C000196266

*To:*_____

*From:*_____

THE WHOLE HEART OF

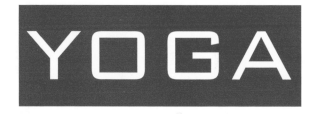

YOGA

THE COMPLETE ORAL TEACHINGS OF THE INDIAN MUSIC MASTERS

CRANE HILL
PUBLISHERS

The Whole Heart of™ *Yoga*
Copyright © 2008 by Fey Family Wu-Su, Inc.

Book design by Pat Covert
Illustrations by Charles D. Fechter Jr.
All calligraphy by Rev. John Bright-Fey

NewForestWay.com

All rights reserved. No part of this book may be reproduced in any form or by
any electronic or mechanical means, including information storage and retrieval
systems, without written permission from the publisher.

"The Whole Heart of" is a trademark of Crane Hill Publishers, Inc.
New Forest® is a registered trademark of Fey Family Wu-Su, Inc.

ISBN-13: 978-1-57587-281-0
ISBN-10: 1-57587-281-1

Printed in China

Library of Congress Cataloging-in-Publication Data

Bright-Fey, J. (John).
   The whole heart of yoga : selected teachings from the original sutras /
John Bright-Fey.
      p. cm.
   ISBN 978-1-57587-281-0
   1. Yoga. I. Title.

B132.Y6B7225 2007
181'.45–dc22

2007043537

THE WHOLE HEART OF

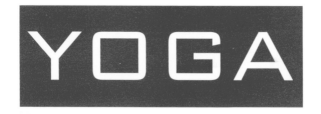

YOGA

THE COMPLETE ORAL TEACHINGS OF THE INDIAN MUSIC MASTERS

REVEREND VENERABLE
JOHN BRIGHT-FEY

CRANE HILL
PUBLISHERS

DEDICATION

In Loving Memory
Howard Roberts
"HR"
Jazz Great, Mentor, Friend

You are missed every single day.

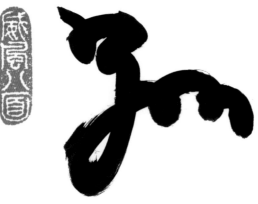

Jhana / Knowledge

TABLE OF CONTENTS

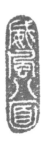 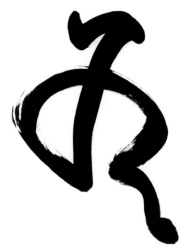

Karma / Active Momentum

THE WHOLE HEART
OF YOGA

This translation is designed to be a study manual that will support a lifetime of involvement in both Hatha Yoga and the practice of Mystic Music. To be sure, it focuses upon the tradition of the Indian Music Masters. But Yoga practitioners will find fresh perspective and a wealth of new information on the practice of their craft as well.

These Sutras are the work of the philosopher-saint known as Patanjali, the founder of Yoga. Precious little is known about this second century BCE Indian mystic, but the impact of his creation continues to affect the world positively.

Both the translation and my comments respond well to transliteration. For example, when you read "song" or "Raga" you may think "posture" or "yoga routine." "To play" means "to perform yoga poses" and "musical instrument" refers to the bodymind of the Hatha Yogi or Yogini.

But there is a more important message within the presentation of this version of Patanjali's Sutras. By seeing precisely how musicians of India's past fused the practice of Yoga with music, you will learn how to unite Yoga with any endeavor. Painting, sculpting, woodworking, dance, cooking, or commerce—literally, anything that human beings do can, and should, be approached yogically. A life fully informed and supported by the "music of yoga" or the "yoga of music" is a life that both nourishes and is nourishing. It illuminates and shapes. It is, at once, something beautiful and something that creates beauty.

The Verse

Each chapter, or aphorism, is presented in verse form, as I received it. No written text was involved in the transmission. I was encouraged to listen to the words and repeat what had been spoken. I was then required to express each aphorism musically and allow the experience to refine the verse. The choices of English poetic structure are my own and reflect the long hours of oral recitation necessary to memorize these Sutras. Each aphorism of a Sutra is a sophisticated condensation of precept and knowledge. This is a hallmark of oral wisdom traditions. All pertinent information is reduced to its utmost limit. Nothing extra is included. Following the verse will be my commentary and instruction. This is divided into four areas:

Mind: This section will contain my exposition into the dynamics of each aphorism. Within the tradition of Indian Music Masters, the translation of the Sutra is all important. Taking each as an object of meditation forms the bulk of the mystic's contemplative study. With time, necessary wisdom is expected to manifest. This wisdom takes the form of flashes of intuitive insight, mystic visions, emotions, and physical sensations. It is quite beyond ordinary intellectual investigation. In fact, many Gurus will simply not explain them in any way, leaving it to the student to contemplate and decipher. In this edition, however, I will attempt to detail the most salient points in each Sutra chapter within this section.

Body: This section will explain how to apply the aphorism in your day-to-day existence. Aligning your behavior with the wisdom of an aphorism entails changing your habits and challenging your preconceptions about life, living, and other people. This requires the ability to, in many ways, face your own dissolution. Deconstructing your normal self and embracing your true self is the task to which every mystic musician is dedicated. Think of these as recipes for living a life guided by the philosophy of Patanjali.

Hand: This section will include the mystic practices that form the basis of a complete understanding of the Sutras. An aphorism cannot be thoroughly understood by the intellect alone. Within the esoteric music tradition, each of Patanjali's aphorisms must be mystically unlocked before the complete force and knowledge contained within is revealed.

To that end, each aphorism is associated with a specific Yoga *asana* (pose) and a *dhyana* (meditation). Asana practice vitalizes the experience of the aphorism and reveals its energy. Dyhana stabilizes the aphorism within the consciousness so it may be thoroughly contemplated and intuitively opened. Practicing one or both of these techniques while comtemplating the aphorism reveals the true knowledge contained within each aphorism. This approach—completely revealed for the first time—represents a secret teaching of the Indian Music Masters.

The specific dhyana technique for each aphorism is presented in the form of a Yoga dhyana meditation. For example, here is the meditation for the fourteenth aphorism of the first Sutra:

Yoga Dhyana Meditation: Asana: **Butterfly Pose**; Mudra: **Lotus**; Chakra: **7th Sahasrara**; Visualize: **Lotus-flower shape and rainbow colors**; Mantram: **Hum**.

This formula is interpreted in this way: **Sit in Butterfly Pose** and form the **Lotus Mudra** with your hands and arms. Rest your mind on the **seventh**, or **Sahasrara Chakra**. Visualize a **Lotus-flower shape** or the **colors of the rainbow** at the top of your head. You may silently intone the **Mantram "Hum"** to move deeply within your bodymind. Breathe naturally and comfortably while contemplating the aphorism and allow its hidden meaning to reveal itself.

The meditation formulas for all of the aphorisms in this volume are interpreted in the same way.

Author's Note: I will assume that the reader has a working knowledge of Hatha Yoga postures. That having been said, it is not absolutely necessary. During the time of Patanjali almost all Yoga was *Raja* (Royal), that is, meditative Yoga. The technique of employing asana to vitalize the experience of each aphorism evolved later and became an integral part of the Indian Music Master's teaching method.

Heart: This section will present each aphorism's core principles. Within esoteric music circles, success comes when the whole heart of an aphorism, that is its essence, is mystically grasped. While study is taking place, a Music Master will drop hints to the student and give clues as to the true meaning behind the words of the aphorism. It is even considered dangerous to understand certain passages too quickly. To that end—and to paraphrase Dickinson—a Music Master will endeavor to tell the truth, but tell it slant. I will bow to tradition in this section and provide clues that will help you decipher the esoteric meaning of the aphorisms.

Dhyana Asana, Mudra, and Mantram

In order to fully explore the mysteries of Patanjali's Sutras, meditation techniques specific to each aphorism must be performed. These techniques are specially designed to create subtle mystic states that alter the consciousness. These altered states of consciousness are necessary for a deep penetration into the hidden wisdom of each aphorism. A complete understanding of the Sutras is, quite literally, impossible without them. In addition to the repetition of a mantram, each meditation (or dhyana) requires the formation of a specific body posture (or asana) with a meditative hand posture (or mudra).

Dhyana Asanas: Postures for Meditation

The practice of dhyana (or meditation) in music yoga most often occurs while the yogi holds a static pose. This facilitates quiescence and a high degree of inner focus that is necessary to cultivate the mind, body, and life force energy (or *prana*). This focus is required to engineer the subtle mystic state associated with each aphorism. What follows are the static poses that are used in contemplating each aphorism of Patanjali's Sutras.

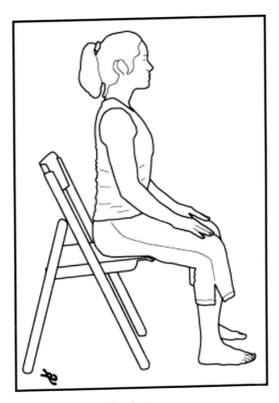

Chair Pose

Sit naturally upright with your feet flat on the floor and palms face down on the knees and thighs. Gently tuck your chin inward, encouraging a lifting feeling at the crown of your head.

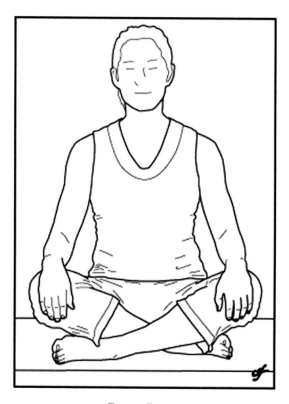

Easy Pose

Sit cross-legged on the ground. If you would like, use a cushion to be more comfortable.

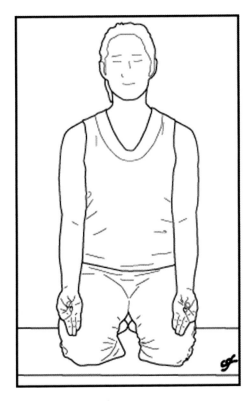

Sitting Pose

This is sometimes called the "Bestriding Rock Posture." Sit upright on your heels with the tops of your feet resting on the ground. Tuck your chin inward. Ideally, your big toes should touch.

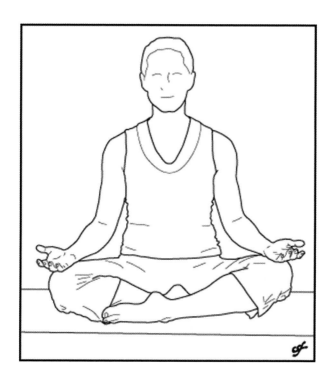

Stability Lotus

Simply cross your legs with both feet touching the ground.

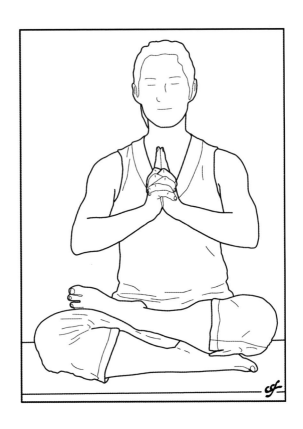

Half-Lotus

Sit cross-legged with one leg on the opposite thigh and the other pulled in tight. Use a cushion, if necessary, to support your top knee.

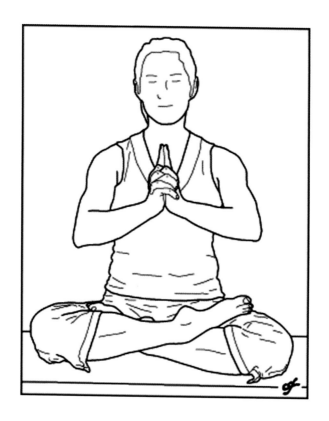

Full Lotus

To form a Full Lotus, sit on the floor with your legs
outstretched in a "V" shape. Bend your left or right knee and
place your foot on top of your opposite thigh as close to
your torso as is comfortable. Bring in the other foot, lifting it
over the first, and place it on top of its opposite thigh.

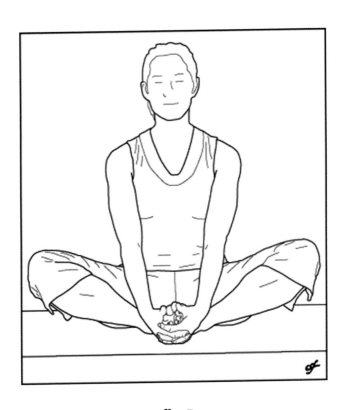

Butterfly Pose

Sit with the soles of your feet touching and pull both of
your heels inward toward your groin. For extra comfort,
it is permissible to put cushions under your knees.

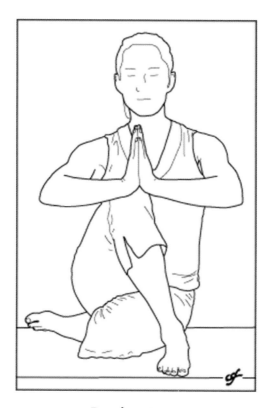

Resting Pose

Sit in Resting Pose by curling one leg under you and placing the opposite leg over it. The top foot should ideally be placed flat on the floor with the knee as upright as is comfortable for you.

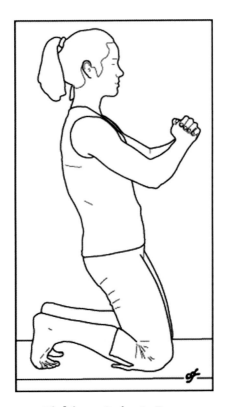

Rishi or Saint's Pose

Rest on your knees and the balls of your feet as shown.
Your right foot and knee should be anywhere from a few
inches up to a foot from your left foot and knee. Lean
backward slightly to complete this pose.

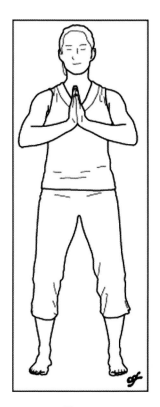

Standing Pose

Stand with your feet parallel and roughly shoulder width apart. Your body weight is shared evenly by your legs.

Dhyana Mudra: Hand Postures For Meditation

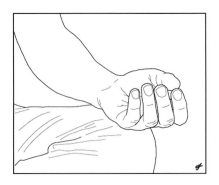

Silent Mudra

Rest the hands on the legs palms up.

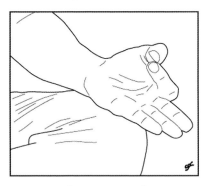

Balance Mudra

Join the first finger and thumb, with the other three fingers extended.

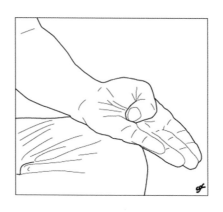

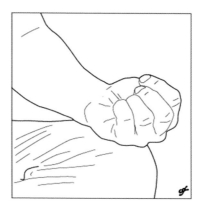

Vitality Mudra

Gently grasp your thumbs with your fingers.

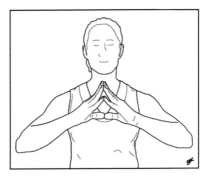

Centering Mudra

Place your hands together, but don't allow the palms to touch. Keep your elbows down and press your fingers and thumbs together.

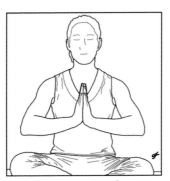

Prayer Mudra

Press your hands together as if gently gluing your palms one to the other.

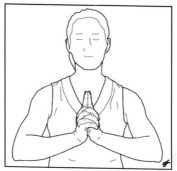

One-Finger Mudra

Interlock the fingers of both hands with the first fingers pointing.

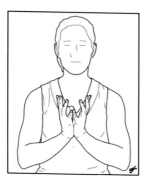

Lotus Mudra

Place the bases of your palms together and hold your fingers outward as though they were the blossoms of a flower.

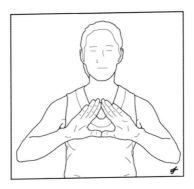

Diamond Mudra

Bring hands together with thumbs and forefingers touching,
forming a triangle. Put subtle strength in your forefingers.

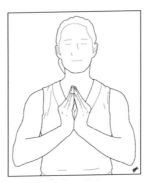

Fire Mudra

Bring your hands together as if to form the shape of a lantern
with a space inside. You may envision an object of
meditation within the space between the hands.

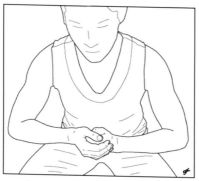

Cosmic Union Mudra

Make a light fist with one hand and cover it with the fingers of the other hand. For men, the left should cover the right; for women, the right should cover the left.

Mantram: Sacred Sounds For Meditation

A mantram (or mantra) is a sound that moves life force energy, expands the consciousness, enhances mental focus, and quiets the mind. Mantrams activate the Chakras which themselves are focal points of energy or prana.

Each Chakra is, among other things, a bridge to a specific level of consciousness and a doorway to subtle realms of existence. Mantrams are the keys that unlock those doors. On the other side is divine song and inspiration that fuels the life of the musician.

The mantrams used in this tradition begin with those that activate the seven Chakra centers of the bodymind. There is some debate in the modern Yoga community regarding the specific location of each Chakra. Indian Music Masters have relied on meditation to reveal the precise location, color, and shape of each Chakra to the fledgling musician. This is an extremely personal process. In this book, I will present general information regarding the Chakras so that your mystical journey may begin on solid footing. That information is included in the text.

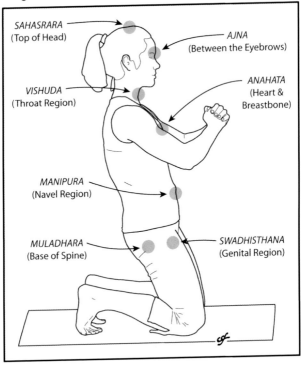

SAHASRARA
(Top of Head)

AJNA
(Between the Eyebrows)

VISHUDA
(Throat Region)

ANAHATA
(Heart &
Breastbone)

MANIPURA
(Navel Region)

MULADHARA
(Base of Spine)

SWADHISTHANA
(Genital Region)

The mantrams and Chakras used for this Whole Heart are:

1) "Lam" for the Muladhara Chakra

2) "Vam" for the Swadhisthana Chakra

3) "Ram" for the Manipura Chakra

4) "Yam" for the Anahata Chakra

5) "Ham" for the Vishuda Chakra
The sound of the first five mantrams is somewhere between an "ahh…" and an "uhh…" sound. Therefore, the mantram "Lam" would sound like, "L…ahh…uhh…mmm" when made with one breath.

6) "Aum" or "Om" for the Ajna Chakra
The sound of "Aum" is actually three sounds that run together, "Aaa…uuu…mmm. It sounds vaguely like "Ow….umm."

7) "Hum" for the Sahasrara Chakra
This sounds like "Whom" in the English language. Some schools of Yoga do not assign a sound to the seventh Chakra. However, within the tradition of Indian Music Masters, "Hum" not only awakens the Sahasrara but connects the player to the music of the Divine.

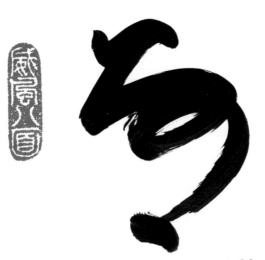

Midha / To Become Invisible

SUTRA BOOK 1

On Learning Mystic Contemplation
Samadhi Pada

This first Sutra is an exposition into the theory of mystic contemplation. It is customary in treatises of this kind to provide an overview of the entire subject to be addressed. Patanjali provides this comprehensive survey in this Sutra.

APHORISM NUMBER 1

**Now herewith begins
An exposition into
The dynamics and inner workings
Of Music Yoga.
Listen with your soul.**

Mind: During the oral transmission process, those in attendance are asked to listen in a thoroughly non-ordinary way. They do this in order to receive the vast spiritual subtext that the Guru is communicating along with the spoken words of the Sutra. This amounts to an act of "metaphysical attending" to a wisdom that exists apart from the limitations of the ordinary world.

Body: Throughout your day, attempt to experience everything you encounter as if it were some wondrous thing you've never seen before. In essence, treat everything like the miracle it truly is. Even when performing common tasks, remember your higher ideals and make yourself transparent to God.

Hand:
- Yoga Asana Posture: Bodhi-asana (Sacred Tree Pose) opens the sixth Chakra and projects prana upwards towards the seventh. This excites the life force to high levels throughout the body and the mind. Spiritually, the perception clears and the ability to mystically hear, feel, and even see music manifests. This state of being is essential for the yogi musician who must rely upon spontaneous intuition to guide his performance.

- Yoga Dhyana Meditation: Asana: **Butterfly Pose**; Mudra: **Lotus**; Chakra: **6th Ajna**; Visualize: **Oval shape or the color blue-gray**; Mantram: **Aum**.

Heart: The secret of this aphorism resides within the spirit of growth, renewal, and creative potential, all of which are vital to the evolution of the mystic musician. Simply put, trust in life's strength, allow it to enter you completely, and be open to the change it fosters. The rest will take care of itself.

APHORISM NUMBER 2

**The essence of Yoga
Rests upon the act of
Innocent restraint
That inhibits any alteration
Of the true mind.**

Mind: The fundamental concept of Yoga revolves around the image of a pool of water. When the surface of the pool is left undisturbed and in its natural state, it is able to reflect things as they really are. This is the "true mind." However, when the surface of the pool is disturbed, the reflected image becomes distorted. It, then, presents a false picture of reality. The work of yoga centers upon restraining those things that disturb the surface of the pool. The idea of innocence reflects a desire to gently inhibit alterations of the true mind with an unforced purity. This concept is fundamental to mystic musicianship.

Body: Setting the stage for a complete understanding of both this aphorism and those that follow begins by doing your best to develop a sharp mind and the ability to reason clearly. Develop independence and efficiency in your daily affairs. Avoid cynicism and cultivate a benevolent spirit.

Hand:
- Yoga Asana Posture: Sav-asana (Corpse Pose) sets the stage for a deeper understanding of this aphorism.

- Yoga Dhyana Meditation: Asana: **Chair, Stability, or Lotus posture;** Mudra: **Silent;** Chakra: **1st Muladhara;** Visualize: **Square shape or the colors yellow and gold**; Mantram: **Laam**.

Heart: The heart of this aphorism lies within the mystical region of your essential experience of life. Authentic Yoga is not created or even practiced. Rather, it is found—composed, really—amid those personal insights and realizations that give you strength and nourishment. Authentic Yogic emancipation must begin with personal renewal. For that renewal to take place you must first plunge into your own experience with abandon and embrace whatever you find there.

APHORISM NUMBER 3

**The Seer of the True Mind
Establishes
His authenticity and
Reveals
His essential nature.**

**Thus, it becomes his foundation
And silent song of emancipation.**

Mind: This aphorism clearly states the result of following the instructions contained in Patanjali's Sutra. The idea of a silent song of emancipation, also known as the Pure and Silent Song, is common among mystic musicians. It underscores the notion that true realization can only be grasped within and not understood from without.

Body: Encourage peaceful relationships wherever you go. Embrace profound relaxation. Be thoughtful and fair in all of your interactions with others as you work to resolve conflicts as you find them. Balance your workday with an equal amount of leisure and repose.

Hand:
- Yoga Asana Posture: Bal-asana (Child's Pose) lays the foundation for unlocking this aphorism.

- Yoga Dhyana Meditation: Asana: **Chair, Stability, or Lotus posture**; Mudra: **Silent**; Chakra: **2nd Swadhisthana**; Visualize: **Upturned crescent shape or the color silver**; Mantram: **Vam**.

Heart: The peace achieved by surrendering to the Yogic process is the key to understanding the mystic heart of this aphorism. The emphasis, of course, rests with the authenticity of your experience. Sham peacefulness in the absence of a balanced and harmonious life results in implacability that blocks any achievement in Yoga.

APHORISM NUMBER 4

In false states of awareness
The Seer is cut off
From the Pure and Silent Song
And allows himself to be shaped and changed
By the alterations
That obscure the True Mind.

Mind: The thoughts you think, your actions, and the words you use all have consequences. In this case the consequence is a life, body, mind, and spirit fundamentally altered according to an illusion created by the alterations of the True Mind. Think of these alterations as corrupted software that finds its way onto a computer. At first, the corrupted software impedes the normal function of the computer, causing its system to operate slowly and even periodically crash. Eventually, the software begins to affect the hardware by actually changing the molecular structure, shape, and appearance of the computer. While fantastic from a modern perspective, Patanjali plainly states that modifications of the True Mind alter both soma and psyche; that is, the body as well as the mind.

Body: Self-observation is the warp and woof of Yoga. Observe the language you use when speaking to others and, more importantly, to yourself. These words color your entire experience. How do you identify yourself to others? Do you call yourself "doctor" or "artist?" Do you see things from a limited or pessimistic perspective? How often do you embrace certitude with your words and actions? For example, phrases like, "All dogs are mean" will cause you to react with fear at the sight (or thought) of any dog no matter how docile or inoffensive. During the day, ask yourself how your words, thoughts, and habits affect your experience. Contrary to the old chestnut, seeing isn't believing. In truth, we are only able to see what we already believe.

Hand:
- Yoga Asana Posture: Bilik-asana (Cat Pose) will set the stage for a complete understanding of this aphorism.

- Yoga Dhyana Meditation: Asana: **Lotus, Stability, or Easy pose**; Mundra: **Vitality**; **2nd Swadhisthana**; Visualize: **Upturned crescent shape and the colors silver and white**; Mantram: **Vam**.

Heart: The secret to fully understanding this aphorism lies with the reconciliation of thought achieved through fair and balanced self-observation. You must see yourself as a full partner with eternity. Together, you and eternity must learn to ride through time creating harmony, peace, and enjoyment wherever you go.

APHORISM NUMBER 5

These alterations that obscure
The True Mind,
Manifest in five different ways
And are experienced as
Ushering in the pain of dissonance or
Ushering in the peace of harmony.

Mind: *Vritti* are the alterations of the mind-substance that frame and delineate the True Mind. These *Vritti*, which are about to be explained in the following aphorisms, ultimately bring pain (*Klista*) or peace (*Aklista*) to the yogi. These are sophisticated concepts. Other pairs of words that may help you to grasp their depth of meaning are unkind and kind, greedy and giving, afflicted and non-afflicted, selfish and selfless, cruel and kind, life-negating and life-affirming. The ideas of pleasure, comfort, satisfaction, and happiness are not necessarily part of the process. A situation that begins as pleasurable, for example, can end in great pain and discomfort. Likewise, an experience, such as a healing trauma, can begin as very painful but eventually ushers in a state of peaceful health and wellness.

Body: Recognize the interconnectedness of your life with the life all around you. Be intuitive throughout your day and engage a holistic perspective whenever possible. Now is the time to engage in teamwork and innovative thinking. In doing so, you will begin to resonate with the wisdom of this aphorism.

Hand:
- Yoga Asana Posture: Ustra-asana (Camel Pose) engages and stimulates the intuition necessary to fully comprehend the depths of this aphorism.

- Yoga Dhyana Meditation: Asana: **Lotus Pose, Stability Pose, or Easy Pose**; Mudra: **One-Finger**; Chakra: **5th Vishuda**; Visualize: **Circle shape or the color white**; Mantram: **Ham**.

Heart: To understand the mystic heart of this aphorism is to fully understand the true meaning of revolution. Too often we equate progress, objectivity, and intelligence with thinking and theorizing. Smashing pre-existing paradigms usually follows this process. Unfortunately, the eternal truth is concealed in the pre-existing reality that is already before us. The secret of this aphorism resides with our ability to allow the eternal to emerge from what we find in front of us. It awaits each of us to call it forth without force or coercion.

APHORISM NUMBER 6

**The five waves of thought
That wash over the consciousness are:
Valid knowledge,
Delusion by misconception,
Flights of verbal fancy,
Dreams, and
Memories.**

Each of these has a sound
That veils the Absolute.

Mind: In this aphorism, Patanjali lists the five kinds of waves that can disturb the surface of the yogic pool. Translators often use the phrase "wrong knowledge" to describe delusion by misconception. This serves to inject a prejudice that, I feel, should be avoided in any discussion of the five alterations. These fluctuations that continuously wash across our consciousness arise within us and are neither good nor bad, nor right or wrong; they simply "are."

Body: Throughout the day, trust in your own abilities and only engage in activity that fosters deep meaning for you. Avoid arrogance at all costs and do not force your ideas on others. Above all, cultivate an abiding trust in God. It is important to note that at the time of Patanjali all vital Yoga was primarily Yoga of the mind. That having been said, how ordinary activity was performed figured greatly into the yogi's quest for emancipation.

Hand:
• Yoga Asana Posture: Surya Namaskar (Sun Salutation) moves life force energy throughout the bodymind and equally stimulates and supports the function of all seven Chakra. It will prepare you for discovering the hidden meaning of this aphorism.

• Yoga Dhyana Meditation: Asana: **Standing Pose**; Mudra: **Prayer**; Chakra: **2nd Swadhisthana**;

Visualize: **Upturned crescent shape or the colors silver and white**; Mantram: **Vam**.

Heart: The secret to grasping the whole heart of this aphorism is to eschew your own separateness from the rest of the world. You are past, present, and future. You must absorb that notion of discovery in which you simultaneously see yourself as both a native of your country and a citizen of the Universe.

APHORISM NUMBER 7

**Valid knowledge
Comes from
Direct contact,
Direct inference, and
Direct testimony by trusted sources.**

Mind: In this case, valid knowledge is acquired when you come into direct contact with an event in spacetime. The organs of preception, or sense organs, relay information—via the central nervous system—to the organ of perception we know as the brain. Valid knowledge is also acquired through sound reasoning based upon the data supplied by direct contact. In this case it is called indirect valid knowledge. For example, you see a Postal vehicle pull up in front of your house. (This is valid knowledge resulting from direct contact.) Based upon past experience, you reason that the Postal carrier might bring you a letter. (This is valid knowledge based on inference.) Before you go to the mailbox, your next-door neighbor calls on the phone and tells you that he just saw the carrier put a letter into your mailbox. (This is an example of valid knowledge resulting from direct testimony.) It should be noted that in ancient yogic thought all "testimony by trusted sources" came from either the reading or recitation of sacred scripture or the utterances of a mystic in the throes of a trance.

Body: Learn how to touch, listen to, and look at the life you encounter with your entire bodymind. Observe all things as if you are astonished at what is transpiring. Endeavor to conduct your affairs in a deliberate and mindful way. Engineering a complete experience of all phenomena is a vital part of the yoga path.

Hand:
- Yoga Asana Posture: Marichy-asana (Sage Twist) helps usher in a complete understanding of this aphorism.

- Yoga Dhyana Meditation: Asana: **Butterfly Pose or Easy Pose**; Mudra: **Centering**; Chakra: **6th Ajna**; Visualize: **Oval shape or the color blue-gray**; Mantram: **Aum.**

Heart: The secret of this aphorism can only be glimpsed at the darkest point of your own personal journey. It is essential that you penetrate the illusion of life and death with your practice so that your unique place amid space and time will be revealed to you. Remember, your goal is not to control the flux and flow of the primal substance that makes up the Universe. Rather, it is your goal to "enter the wilderness" and seek to exercise control over

42

your own consciousness and "still the surface of the pool." Seeing yourself as a unique phenomenon is the key to accomplishing your goal.

APHORISM NUMBER 8

Delusion by misconception
Is intellectual knowledge.
It occurs
When our mental impression
Of a thing
Does not accurately reflect
Its real form.

Hence, the song is falsely conceived.

Mind: This Vritti is called *Viparyaya* and is likened to a mirage, a false perception, or some other misconception. To the yogi this is flawed knowledge that occurs because of lack of information and the rush to judgment. Distortions occur when we rely upon past experience in the absence of present awareness. Indeed, our habits and preconceptions shape our experience of all we perceive.

Body: Embrace new experiences as a way of delving into the meaning of this aphorism. Be bold and open up to something completely different. Change your habitual ways of thinking and reacting. At the very least, break up your everyday routine.

Hand:

- Yoga Asana Posture: Mudra-asana (Psychic Union Pose) helps usher in a complete understanding of this aphorism.

- Yoga Dhyana Meditation: Asana: **Stability Lotus Pose or Easy Pose**; Mudra: **Centering**; Chakra: **3rd Manipura**; Visualize: **Downward-pointed triangle or the color red**; Mantram: **Raam**.

Heart: The secret of this aphorism will be found at that sacred point where the real and the false nature of phenomenal experience meet. Whether a person, place, event, or thing, this is the point where the energy of the moment pulls at you from all directions. This is a pivot point that occurs before any intellectual knowledge is conceived. If you can glimpse this point, then you will glimpse the true mind and "still the surface of the pond." When you begin to feel physically condensed, you will know that your contemplation is about to bear fruit.

APHORISM NUMBER 9

**Imaginative flights of fancy
Occur when spoken or written words
Give rise to images
That have no basis in reality.
This is called verbal delusion.**

Mind: This Vritti is called *Vikalpa*. Delusion by misconception, as discussed in the previous aphorism, requires exposure to some kind of objective data. This exposure, being incomplete, leads you to make a false conclusion about what is being experienced. Vikalpa, on the other hand, occurs without any data being experienced. It is truly a subjective experience. Reading a novel or overhearing a partial conversation and drawing conclusions from what you have read or heard, lead you down the path of verbal delusion.

Body: Engage in enjoyable and relaxing pursuits as a way of putting verbal delusion to route. Flights of fancy may also be neutralized by the realization that the True Mind is abundant, transcendent, and infinite.

Hand:
• Yoga Asana Posture: Virabhadra-Asana (Warrior Pose) prepares you to understand the deeper meaning of verbal delusion as discussed in this aphorism. This posture expands the aura while extending prana outward away from the bodymind. Indian musicians use this posture to build a sheath of life force energy that protects the spirit as well as the body. This allows the musician to freely express himself.

• Yoga Dhyana Meditation: Asana: **Resting Pose, Butterfly Pose, or Easy Pose**; Mudra: **Prayer**; Chakra: **6th Ajna**; Visualize: **Oval shape or the colors blue and gray**; Mantram: **Aum**.

Heart: To understand the nature of verbal delusion and eventually gain control over it requires a connectedness to the earth that reveals the truth of your terrestrial existence. It also requires insight into the cycle of birth and death with regards to that existence.

APHORISM NUMBER 10

When the confused sights and sounds of nothingness
That occur during sleep
Alter and modify the consciousness
It is called the music of dreaming.

Mind: For yogi in the Indian music tradition, the field of dreams is a dimension of sacred sound and song that flows from the heart of Eternity. But eternity does not possess a quality of time-that-passes. Rather, it is the ripples upon the surface of the True Mind that imposes time and separates us from the ever present dimension of the eternal song. When we dream during sleep, we extend ourselves into this realm and experience the continuous outpouring of dream music, though we have a difficult time making sense of it. Understanding the dynamics of this dream music helps the yogi to still the mind.

Body: Reach out into phenomenal existence. That is, touch as much life as you can. Keeping a dream journal aids in ordering the thought processes. Upon awakening, simply record your dreams or thoughts and impressions about your dreams in a journal. Over time, the sacred dream music will both become clearer and alter the mind less.

Hand:

- Yoga Asana Posture: Performing Surya Namaskar, or Sun Salutation, illuminates the mind to the realities and wonders of the dream realm. Ancient yogis referred to asana not as "postures," but as "dreams" and "memories."

- Yoga Dhyana Meditation: Asana: **Standing Pose**; Mudra: **Lotus**; Chakra: **4th Anahata**; Visualize: **6-pointed star shape or the color light blue**; Mantram: **Yam**.

Heart: The key to comprehending the heart of this aphorism lies in the acceptance of one's own transience. It is the paradox of time-that-passes colliding with the ever-present force of eternity that will reveal it to you. Realize that every night as you go to sleep and every morning as you awake, you are at a turning point. This point, which is fundamentally transformative, allows you to ascend to a new life if you would but take the next step.

APHORISM NUMBER 11

Memories
Alter and modify the consciousness
When past experiences are
Called up and
Held onto.

Mind: Memories retained as deep impressions on the mindscape do not, themselves, cause alterations of the consciousness. The alterations occur when the impressions are summoned to the surface of the mindscape through prolonged recollection. When the surfaced impressions become active through recollection in the immediate waking consciousness, then they cause alterations and modifications.

Body: Above all, be joyful and warmhearted in all of your dealings with others. Extending deep affection and spiritual nourishment wherever you go will help you to embody the esoteric wisdom of this aphorism.

Hand:
• Yoga Asana Posture: Performing the Heart Pose, or Anahata-asana, will guide you towards a complete understanding of this aphorism. Like the meditation that follows, it will activate the energy of belonging and foster a sense of yourself as a member of the universal family. Remember, ancient yogis referred to asana not as "postures," but as "dreams" and "blissful memories."

• Yoga Dhyana Meditation: Asana: **Half-Lotus or Stability Lotus Pose**; Mudra: **Prayer**; Chakra: **4th Anahata**; Visualize: **6-pointed star shape or the color light blue**; Mantram: **Yam**.

Heart: Uncover your carefree and original potential and you will seize the whole heart of this aphorism. It resides in the awareness of the free-flowing characteristics and impermanence of memory. It is this characteristic itself that is a reflection of the True Mind.

**Control of this dissonance
Is accomplished through the practices of
Persistent force of will and
Mindful non-attachment.**

Mind: "Persistent force of will" refers to a precise application of willpower to the task of yogic cultivation. Specifically, it relates to a discipline that fosters authenticity. In the music tradition, for example, one note played with authentic feeling and emotion is considered superior to a dazzling display of many notes that are contrived or overly complex. Within the ancient hatha Yoga culture, only three asana were considered necessary to achieve total emancipation. Yet, modern yoga abounds with practitioners who are invested in practicing many postures. A precise application of effort and willpower opts for a more deliberate and focused approach where the breadth and depth of a simple practice is expanded to include the totality of the adherent's life. To be mindfully non-attached is to approach this expanded discipline in an unhurried manner while allowing it to unfold naturally without interference.

Body: Availing yourself of any opportunity to be pleasantly astonished, happy, and blissful will align your day-to-day life with the wisdom of this aphorism.

Hand:
• Yoga Asana Posture: Ustra-asana (Camel Pose) will align the bodymind with the wisdom of this aphorism.

• Yoga Dhyana Meditation: Asana: **Full Lotus, Stability Lotus, or Easy Pose**; Mudra: **One-Finger**; Chakra: **5th Vishuda**; Visualize: **White circle**; Mantram: **Ham**.

Heart: The secret of this aphorism can only be grasped when you open up completely to the continuously unfolding mystery of universal love that connects all of existence. Once opened up, all that remains is to bring an artistic aesthetic to your practice as a means of exposing the whole heart of the aphorism.

APHORISM NUMBER 13

Of these two methods,
The practice of persistent force of will
Brings self-possessed
Stability of consciousness.

Mind: Another way of translating this aphorism would be:

Of these two methods,
The disciplined practice of authenticity
Ushers in a steadfast, serene, and unfluctuating
State of mind, as well as
An unbroken field of consciousness.

Body: Living one's life in a spontaneous and authentic manner supports the wisdom of this aphorism.

Hand:
- Yoga Asana Posture: Cultivating Settu bandha-asana (Bridge Pose) is said to increase the levels of compassion, spiritual strength, and intuition necessary to grasp the full meaning of this aphorism.

- Yoga Dhyana Meditation: Asana: **Full Lotus, Stability Lotus, or Easy posture**; Mudra: **One-finger**; Chakra: **5th Vishuda**; Visualize: **Circle shape and the color white**; Mantram: **Ham**.

Heart: When on the yoga path, it is vital to avoid forcing your progress. It is the function of Yoga to take the wisdom of *Patanjali* from the realm of words to the realm of direct experience. Cultivate a sense of wholeness and trust in your own abilities.

APHORISM NUMBER 14

When
Over a long time
Spiritual practice is held
Continuously and reverently,
It becomes firmly established
In the ground of being.

Thus,
The authentic Song of Perfect Mastery
Unfolds.

Mind: In this tradition of mystical musicianship, authenticity is the result of activity that is at once natural, spontaneous, disciplined, and planned. Said another way, authenticity arises as a result of organized and deliberate action. This action is so well trained that it takes on an entirely different dimension: it becomes new. Awash in this newness, the yogi, as well as the musician, experiences the infinite.

Body: Avoid aimless activity. Endeavor to turn an idea or project into reality while also securing what you have already achieved. Seeing a task that presents itself, rolling up your sleeves, and tackling it will put you in touch with the spirit of this aphorism.

Hand:
- Yoga Asana Posture: Vrksa-asana (Tree Pose) reveals the inner secret of this aphorism. Regular practice sharpens the senses by drawing prana from deep within the earth and moving it upward through your bodymind. Once this prana is focused, it opens and fortifies the sixth and seventh Chakras.

- Yoga Dhyana Meditation: Asana: **Butterfly Pose**; Mudra: **Lotus**; Chakra: **7th Sahasrara**; Visualize: **Lotus-flower shape or the colors of the rainbow**; Mantram: **Hum**.

Heart: The heart of this aphorism resides in following your individual spiritual path and not one dictated by others. Spiritual independence reminds us that we are unique expressions of the Universe and must be guided by our own higher ideals. Only then will our spiritual practice be stable. Only then will we hear the song of perfect mastery. Said simply, play your song, not someone else's.

APHORISM NUMBER 15

The Song of Perfect Mastery
Manifests in one
Who is unmoved
By those things seen and unseen.

This is mindful non-attachment;
Life without endless craving or color.

Mind: Finding the immovable center within virtually requires the yogi to move beyond any framework in their life that is too narrow and restrictive. This includes, but is not limited to, habitual ways of thinking and behaving. This brings with it all manner of temptations, distractions, dangers, and risks. Ultimately, salvation and liberation await those who can weather the "chaotic storm of sound, shape, and color." The Song of Perfect Mastery refers to the impetus of moving towards the Pure and Silent Song of the Absolute. It also indicates alignment towards that goal.

Body: Seek situations in your day-to-day life that are fundamentally nourishing. At the same time, put your normal routine into a spin and encourage new patterns to emerge.

Hand:
- Yoga Asana Posture: Cultivate Upavistha kona-asana (Seated Angle Pose) as a means of fully understanding the mysteries of this aphorism.

- Yoga Dhyana Meditation: Asana: **Sitting Pose**; Mudra: **Centering**; Chakra: **2nd Swadhisthana**; Visualize: **Upturned crescent shape or the color silver**; Mantram: **Vam**.

Heart: The secret of this aphorism resides at the one unmovable center that lay within all of us. Playfully search it out while relying heavily upon your intuition to guide you.

APHORISM NUMBER 16

**When the Seer
Neither thirsts nor desires
Even the fundamental qualities
Of the natural world,
He reaches supreme non-attachment
And the True Mind manifests.**

Mind: Mystic musicians attempt to connect with the wisdom of this aphorism by playing their music in a soft and subtle manner. At the same time they try to bring an active and forceful quality to it. Each note "should possess both lightness and heaviness." This is a perfect formula for governing all thought and action while experiencing the phenomenal world. It leads to an unmovable state of consciousness that reveals the True Mind.

Body: Traditionally, Masters have encouraged their disciples to support a righteous yet unpopular cause as a means of identifying with the wisdom in this aphorism.

Hand:
• Yoga Asana Posture: Sav-asana (Corpse Pose) reconnects you to your own innocence that, ultimately, establishes the foundation for the liberation, or moksa, of your soul.

• Yoga Dhyana Meditation: Asana: **Chair Pose or Lotus Pose**; Mudra: **Silent**; Chakra: **1st Muladhara**; Visualize: **Square shape or the colors yellow and gold**; Mantram: **Lam**.

Heart: The key to unlocking the whole heart of this aphorism is, simply put, courage.

APHORISM NUMBER 17

Sit and listen.
Attend the Raga;
Rest.

In the beginning,
Four tones emerge from the resting.
The first sounds harsh and shrill;

It judges.
The second sounds melodic and moves definitively;
It reveals.
The third sounds harmonious as it floats here and there;
It equalizes.
The fourth tone settles like dew on morning grass;
It outlines.

Mind: In this translation, "Raga" is synonymous with "song" and "composition." A Seer, or mystic musician, stands with one foot in the consensual realm and one foot in the eternal. His instrument—be it a sitar, tabla, violin, or piano—serves as a compass that constantly seeks the transcendent. The resting mentioned in this aphorism is the act of totally surrendering to a musical composition whether the Seer plays it or hears it. If properly attended to the musical composition will point to the total mystery of life known as the Brahman or God. The Seer must surrender to song.

Body: Any activity that fosters a deep connection with the life around you will support the wisdom of this aphorism.

Hand:
• Yoga Asana Posture: Forming the Adho mukha svan-asana II, or Downward-facing Dog II (also known as the Three-Legged Dog posture), will set the stage for contemplative listening described in this aphorism.

- Yoga Dhyana Meditation: Asana: **Kneeling Pose**;
  Mudra: **Diamond**; Chakra: **7th Sahasrara**;
  Visualize: **Lotus-flower shape or the colors of
  the rainbow**; Mantram: **Hum**.

Heart: The heart of this aphorism resides in the sacred
feminine. Your ability to step back and acquiesce to the
energy of the moment will allow you to see past yourself.

APHORISM NUMBER 18

**As resting continues,
These tones fade away to their source
And rejoin the vast collection
Of unplayed *Raga*
That lay sleeping deep within.
Following the tones to their source
Stills the mind of the Seer.**

Mind: Following the tones to their source engineers a
gradual returning to the domain of the Pure and Silent
Song. Contemplative listening of this kind is of
tremendous value when attempting to still the surface of
the pond. As a continuation of the previous aphorism this
method is one of acquiescence that leads to quiescence.

Body: During the course of your day listen to the sounds
around you. Envision them to be the most beautiful music
you have ever heard. As you take notice of the sounds,
try to follow them and "see" where they go. Listening as
the sounds fade away will generate the increasing levels

of mental clarity needed to grasp the full force of this aphorism.

Hand:
- Yoga Asana Posture: Adho mukha sav-asana, also known as Downward-facing Corpse Pose, helps capture the spirit of this aphorism. It fortifies the energetic body, calms the spirit, and focuses the mind.

- Yoga Dhyana Meditation: Asana **Chair Pose**; Mudra: **Silent**; Chakra: **1st Muladhara**; Visualize: **Square shape or the colors yellow and gold**; Mantram: **Lam**.

Heart: The whole heart of this aphorism resides in the process of surrendering, or to be more precise, sacrificing the ego to the relationship between you and your music or yoga practice.

APHORISM NUMBER 19

**In truth, we are only music.
There is such an abundance of music in each of us
That it can confuse us and complicate things.
It binds us to the manifested;
It separates us from the unmanifested.
But the Pure and Silent Song brings forth
Only the music
Which is of use to each of us.**

To find that one unique Raga
That is within you
Is the key.

Mind: Divinity is our essence. Unfortunately, we become confused and attached to the sheer amount of manifested life—and the possibilities of that life—all around us. This confusion binds us to the consensual and separates us from our spiritual ground of being. Music, more than anything else, has the power to eliminate this confusion.

The notion of one unique song that will lead each of us back to a full realization of our divinity is ubiquitous within the community of mystical musicians. Indeed, our spiritual nourishment and realization depend on it.

Body: Try to see the light of God shining through each person you meet, even those whose behavior you find morally reprehensible.

Hand:
• Yoga Asana Posture: Forming the Janu-sirsa-asana, or Head-to-knee Pose, facilitates a turning inward necessary to find the music within.

• Yoga Dhyana Meditation: Asana: **Sitting Pose**; Mudra: **Balance**; Chakra: **3rd Manipura**; Visualize: **Triangle shape or the color red**; Mantram: **Ram**.

Heart: The secret to discovering the whole heart of this aphorism rests solely in your ability to recognize your personal errors in judgment and precisely how those errors have led to disappointment in your life.

APHORISM NUMBER 20

**Many cannot hear their unique song
So they delight in the expression of others
Instead of their own.
For them
A different way is necessary.
But that way is not as free
And the Seer seeks only freedom.**

Mind: Patanjali plainly states that the path of the Seer isn't for everyone. However, all humanity shares a timeless knowledge concerning the Absolute that is already implicit or *a priori*. This knowledge, native to human minds, responds to authentic creation, and, in this case, music. In the next aphorism Patanjali tells us precisely how this response can be engineered.

Body: Spend time listening to music as a contemplative activity. The entire text of the Yoga Sutra serves as a guide for this kind of contemplation.

Hand:
- Yoga Asana Posture: Form the Danda-asana, or Staff (or Rod) Pose, to align your bodymind with this aphorism. Specifically, it clarifies the life force by uniting the prana of the upper and lower parts of the bodymind.

• Yoga Dhyana Meditation: Asana: **Easy Pose**; Mudra: **Balance**; Chakra: **2nd Swadhisthana**; Visualize: **Upturned crescent shape or the color silver**; Mantram: **Vam**.

Heart: Practicing both Danda-asana and the above meditation will help you to stay alert to the workings of the ego. This is the key to unlocking the heart of this aphorism. Observing the self as you navigate the many contrasting situations of your life and devotional practice will fortify your spiritual goals.

APHORISM NUMBER 21

For them,
The Pure and Silent Song of emancipation can be heard
If they attend the music properly.
If they listen with their whole being
Then realization is never far away.

How should they attend the music?
By listening with their souls.

Mind: Any event in spacetime, be it yoga asana, musical expression, or some other aspect of the phenomenal world, can lead to emancipation. Since all of creation is part of the Brahman, we have but to engineer a complete experience of an aspect of the phenomenal world to glimpse our True Mind and reveal the Source.

Body: Listening with your soul and mystically joining with music being played, requires the ability to enter into an intimate relationship with the music. In essence, you must take the Raga as a lover. Look for examples in your daily life to join forces with others and work together toward heartfelt ends.

Hand:

- Yoga Asana Posture: Creating the Baddha kona-asana (Cobbler's Pose) releases negative attachments that stop you from both, listening *to* and listening *with* your soul.

- Yoga Dhyana Meditation: Asana **Half-Lotus Pose or Stability Lotus Pose**; Mudra: **Prayer**; Chakra: **4th Anahata**; Visualize: **6-pointed star shape or the color light blue**; Mantram: **Yam**.

Heart: The secret to comprehending the full meaning of this aphorism is realizing that contemplative listening is a marriage in the truest sense of the word. Experience the music with your heart.

APHORISM NUMBER 22

**Attending the music properly
Involves subtle and complete soul-listening.**

**This is accomplished by tuning oneself to the Raga
And letting its meaning organize
The hidden memories that lay within the shadows**

Of our being.
But not everyone can surrender completely
To the meaning of the Raga
Or the moment of its creation.
They must surrender gradually or they risk
Losing themselves amid cognition.

Mind: The idea of "tuning oneself to the Raga" is fundamental to mystical musicianship. Every Raga has layers of meaning. In effect, each is a metaphor describing the subtleties of the outer world. In order to completely experience either the act of listening or playing, the Seer must come into alignment with the spiritual realm of the inner world. Then, when encountered, the two will vibrate harmoniously together.

For cultivators of Hatha Yoga, the implications are profound. Namely, that one must tune the bodymind to a specific frequency to fully experience the wonders and benefits of an asana.

Body: Bring a sense of creativity to your everyday tasks and obligations. Looking for new ways to do things within the consensual world will help you to tune your soul. Above all, be in the moment. Getting too caught up in the future will throw your inner self out of tune.

Hand:
- Yoga Asana Posture: Parsva-uttana-asana (Sideways Bend Pose) generates feelings of spiritual ease and

comfort. It helps prevent one from becoming lost "amid cognition."

- Yoga Dhyana Meditation: Asana: **Full Lotus Pose, Stability Lotus Pose, or Easy Pose**; Mudra: **One-finger**; Chakra: **4th Anahata**; Visualize: **6-pointed star shape or the color light blue**; Mantram: **Yam**.

Heart: Grasp the whole heart of this aphorism by engaging in ritual and prayer. This will allow your awareness to expand gradually. Any activity that generates a sense of spiritual ease and comfort will support the deeper meaning of this aphorism as well as the mysteries it unveils.

APHORISM NUMBER 23

But if they succeed in opening their being completely,
They will hear the genuine and undiluted sound
Of complete and unbridled experience
That is called *Ishvara*.

Ishvara itself is not the Pure and Silent Song.
Yet, the Pure and Silent Song
Cannot be heard without it.

It is a complete and incomprehensible tone
Residing at the center
Of all music.

Mind: Ishvara is the undiluted and flawless essence of experience. Think of it as a clarified transcendental vibration at the heart of every single thing in the phenomenal world. Historically, mystic musicians have also referred to it as *Naam*, or the "Holy Word."

Body: Cultivating Ishvara during your everyday experience requires a subtle shift in perspective. Rather than thinking of yourself as a physical being engaging in spiritual practice, think of yourself as a spiritual being engaging in physical activity as a way of more deeply understanding the wonders of the Absolute.

Hand:

- Yoga Asana Posture: Creating Bhujang-asana (Cobra Pose) facilitates the profound opening of the entire being as described in this aphorism. It also helps combat feelings of separateness.

- Yoga Dhyana Meditation: Asana: **Easy Pose**; Mudra: **Vitality**; Chakra: **2nd Swadhisthana**; Visualize: **Upturned crescent shape or the color silver**; Mantram: **Vam**.

Heart: The secret of this aphorism is simple: you must acknowledge the truth of your terrestrial connection. While it is true that you are a spiritual being exploring the wonders of the Universe, the motive force for this exploration comes from the Earth itself.

APHORISM NUMBER 24

The true Ishvara is complete
In and of itself
And is connected to all that exists.
Yet, it is also unfettered by all that exists.

It is in every move you make
And all that you see and hear.
It resides in every note of every Raga.
It binds the room together when we play.

Mind: Said another way, every song or asana is connected to every other song or asana. When you *know* one, you *know* them all. Furthermore, it is possible to see a song or an asana at the heart of anything you experience in the world. This world—our world—is held together by the music of Raga and Yoga asana. Mystic musicians feel this unity during prolonged performance or practice sessions.

Body: Standing up for oneself and expressing personal needs conscientiously builds an everyday foundation for accessing the spiritual wisdom contained in this aphorism. Conscientiousness in this case eschews egotistical self-assertion and, instead, embraces mature independence.

Hand:
- Yoga Asana Posture: Sukh-asana, also known as Happy Pose, echoes the mysteries of this aphorism

while engendering a deep Cosmic trust. It also generates the type of joy associated with Ishvara.

- Yoga Dhyana Meditation: Asana: **Easy Pose**; Mudra: **Vitality**; Chakra: **1st Muladhara**; Visualize: **Square shape or the colors yellow and gold**; Mantram: **Lam**.

Heart: The secret of this aphorism and the secret to revealing Ishvara is the same. The whole heart resides in the ability to turn a burning passion for music into the energy of spiritual endeavor.

APHORISM NUMBER 25

**Its transcendental nature
Bestows a uniqueness that exists
Of its own accord.
It accompanies itself and in doing so
Reveals the Absolute.**

**It can be heard only when a Seer
Plays amid timelessness.**

Mind: Revealing the transcendental nature of Ishvara during musical performance is both a goal and a product of authentic musical expression within the mystic context. From that context, it is the function of music to transport us beyond words and ideas to the experience of infinity.

Body: Engaging in activity that promotes emotional flexibility supports the message of this aphorism. Strive to eliminate possessiveness in yourself and cultivate optimism and acceptance when meeting others.

Hand:

- Yoga Asana Posture: The Nataraj-asana, or Shiva Dance Pose, reveals both the timelessness and the transcendental nature of the universe.

- Yoga Dhyana Meditation: Asana: **Resting Pose, Butterfly Pose, or Easy Pose**; Mudra: **Centering**; Chakra: **7th Sahasrara**; Visualize: **Lotus-flower shape or the colors of the rainbow**; Mantram: **Hum**.

Heart: The key to grasping the whole heart of this aphorism can be summed up by the phrase, "bring light into the darkness."

APHORISM NUMBER 26

**Being a timeless Raga,
It has always been the musicians' ideal.
It is the Raga that cannot be explained.
It can only be sought after;
Divined;
Felt.**

Mind: Mystical music within the East Indian tradition is improvisational in nature. The Seer must freely improvise within the delineated confines of a given composition. This includes, but is not limited to, rules defining fixed notes of tension and resolution, procedures that govern the development of overall musical themes, and precepts that determine the time of day a specific Raga can be played. Playing within these limits yields a creative intensity that, in part, engineers the mystical experience. As that experience unfolds, the musician moves through it the same way a dowser searches for water. Intuitively moving from one sensation to another as he plays, the Seer gradually learns to move from the time-bound to the timeless. Eventually, he learns to navigate the web of consciousness that enfolds the planet and our experience of it.

Body: As you go about your day, suggest to yourself that everyone and everything you encounter is, in reality, a part of yourself. There are no boundaries of language, culture or any other division.

Hand:
- Yoga Asana Posture: Create the Paripurma nav-asana (or Kriya-asana), or Longboat Pose, to align yourself with the wisdom of this aphorism. Specifically, it ushers in a general change of vision wherein you see the totality of the world around you.

- Yoga Dhyana Meditation: Asana: **Easy Pose**; Mudra: **Balance**; Chakra: **3rd Manipura**; Visualize: **Triangle shape or the color red**; Mantram: **Ram**.

Heart: Grasping the whole heart of this aphorism begins with the courage to passionately devote yourself to the left-handed path of intuitive exploration. Whether it's a task, an experience, or an individual, being confidently self-guided rather than led reflects the essence of this aphorism.

APHORISM NUMBER 27

The *Tamboura* calls it forth
And puts it within our reach.
It guides us to our Raga and
Tells us how to play.
It is Om;
Our standard,
Our goal,
Our source.

Mind: Om (also aum) is the most enduring and all-embracing symbol in Hinduism. It represents the sum total of spiritual knowledge and the manifestation of its power. Though not a word in the accepted sense, it is a vibration or seed syllable that lies at the center of all words, all matter, and all sound. The Tamboura, a drone instrument that plays in the background of East Indian music, creates a canvas of resonant sound. This resonant sound draws out the vibration Om from deep within the phenomenal realm. The Seer then "paints" his musical improvisation upon the Om canvas and, in doing so, outlines the wonders of the Absolute at work within the ordinary world. Simply put, he shows us God.

Body: Expanding your horizons will put you in touch with the wisdom of this aphorism. Do something new and interesting.

Hand:
- Yoga Asana Posture: Create the Viksa-asana, or Tree Pose, to unlock the mysteries of this aphorism.

- Yoga Dhyana Meditation: Asana: **Butterfly Pose**; Mudra: **Lotus**; Chakra: **7th Sahasrara**; Visualize: **Lotus-flower shape or the colors of the rainbow**; Mantram: **Hum**.

Heart: Unlock the whole heart of this aphorism by eliminating possessiveness and the need to be in control. Above all, avoid being too theoretical and thoughtful. The spiritual and the earthly world penetrate one another. We have but to outline that point of contact to glimpse the wonders of each.

APHORISM NUMBER 28

**The more we play our instrument
The clearer our source becomes.
But this clarity cannot be rushed.
Ishvara finds us
In its own time amid timelessness
And finds us only when we are ready.
It requires great faith and devotion.**

Mind: Lewis Carroll created the word "galumphing" to describe a state of play where the rules are few but the adventures are many. Play in this case is engaging in rambunctious abandon within the confines of the given artistic expression. Expectations are kept to a minimum. In fact, both the musician and the yogi should play without any thought of reward or outcome. Creating the music or asana simply for the sheer pleasure of creation is reason enough. Only then will Ishvara find us.

Body: Attempting to "read between the lines" of normal activity will help you to resonate with the spirit of this aphorism. Look for the subtext of the situations you find yourself in.

Hand:
• Yoga Asana Posture: Adho mukha svanasana (Downward-facing Dog) is designed to clear the perception so we might see the hidden side of life.

• Yoga Dhyana Meditation: Asana **Chair Pose**; Mudra **Vitality**; Chakra: **2nd Swadhisthana**; Visualize: **Upturned crescent shape or the color silver**; Mantram: **Vam**.

Heart: The whole heart of this aphorism resides in your ability to first achieve something of worth or great value. Once it has been achieved, the second step is to allow yourself to thoroughly enjoy it.

When Ishvara does find us,
It is our duty to absorb it completely
So we may ready ourselves to experience the
totality
Of the Pure and Silent Song.

But even as we begin surrendering to it,
Impediments dissolve,
Discriminations cease, and
Walls are breached.

Such is the power of music.
Indeed, nothing is more powerful.

Mind: In the final analysis, all music and all yoga asana are works of art. But we do not create them. Rather, we invite them into our very being so they may temporarily inhabit us. The Seer must open up to the song and meet it on its terms and not his own. Even a small allowing of this kind is a powerful way to still the surface of the pond.

Body: As you go about your day, allow all of your thoughts and actions to be informed with the notion that you are a manifestation of spirit.

Hand:
• Yoga Asana Posture: Vajra-asana (Thunderbolt Pose) mirror the spiritual actions spoken about in this

aphorism. Creating it clears spiritual perception and insight.

- Yoga Dhyana Meditation: Asana: **Resting Pose, Butterfly Pose, or Easy Pose**; Mudra: **Vitality**; Chakra: **6th Ajna**; Visualize: **Oval shape or the color blue-gray**; Mantram: **Aum**.

Heart: Whether asana or music, you must spiritually surrender to the creation of your art. This is the secret to comprehending the aphorism and accessing its hidden meaning.

APHORISM NUMBER 30

Many things can separate us from the Pure and Silent Song.
Your thinking mind stands as a watchman
Between the True and the Deluded self.
You must not allow the wrong things inside.
Particularly, avoid self-indulgence.

Mind: The notion that your thinking mind stands in the breach between truth and delusion is a profound one. Let me be as plain as I am able—what you choose to think about determines the health of your spiritual life. Ultimately, we are in control of what we think about and what we allow to influence us. Yet, for so many people what they think about—and how they think about it—is habitual. Above all, these habitual themes and the manner in which you cognitively interact with them must change if your devotional practice is to be successful.

Body: Whenever you find yourself thinking negatively, purposefully and deliberately focus your thoughts on something positive and uplifting. To be a Seer you must have the ability to deliberately change the thoughts that you think. Make conscious and willful choices about what you choose to see, hear, and, functionally, let into your mind.

Hand:

- Yoga Asana Posture: Creating the Parvsa-kona-asana, or Side Angle Pose, allows us to view the inner workings of the "watchman." This asana is a powerful tool for putting habitually negative thinking to route.

- Yoga Dhyana Meditation: Asana: **Stability Lotus Pose or Easy Pose**; Mudra: **Centering**; Chakra: **3rd Manipura**; Visualize: **Triangle shape or the color red**; Mantram: **Ram**.

Heart: The secret to grasping the whole heart of this aphorism can be found in your ability to purposefully seek happiness and joy. Draw upon all of your emotional and intellectual resources and blissfully enjoy any moment you find yourself in.

APHORISM NUMBER 31

Self-indulgence causes
Illness, loneliness, grief,
And loss of physical control.
It disturbs the breath and
Causes the soul to drift
From its vital center and stillpoint.

Mind: Idly doing what pleases you regardless of the negative consequences to yourself or others blocks the free flow of prana or life force energy throughout your bodymind. The surface of the pond is, likewise, greatly disturbed.

Body: Expressing deep affection for close friends or family will put you in resonance with the wisdom of this aphorism.

Hand:
- Yoga Asana Posture: Sav-asana (Corpse Pose) puts us in touch with the essence of this aphorism. It specifically remedies loneliness and grief, as well as other negative attachments produced by habitual self-indulgence.

- Yoga Dhyana Meditation: Asana: **Chair Pose**; Mudra: **Silent**; Chakra: **1st Muladhara**; Visualize: **Square shape or the colors yellow and gold**; Mantram: **Lam**.

Heart: The key to grasping the whole heart of this aphorism rests in your ability to calmly let situations evolve without your interference or imposed expectations.

APHORISM NUMBER 32

The Seer can overcome these disturbances
By the way he creates his life and
By the way he creates his music.
Indeed, for the true Seer
Life and music are the same.

Mind: How might you think and behave if you created your day-to-day life the same way you create music? Many creatively successful artists have a life that is in constant conflict and shambles. But the mystic musician strives to allow his art to inform his everyday life and vice versa.

Body: Expressing emotional openness and consideration for others will bring your behavior into alignment with this aphorism.

Hand:
• Yoga Asana Posture: Marichy-asana, also known as the Sage Twist, is invaluable in unlocking the wisdom of this aphorism. It is specifically designed to penetrate illusion and reveal your sacred place in spacetime.

• Yoga Dhyana Meditation: Asana: **Resting Pose, Butterfly Pose, or Easy Pose**; Mudra: **Centering**;

Chakra: **6th Ajna**; Visualize: **Oval shape or the color blue-gray**; Mantram: **Aum**.

Heart: How well you bring your professional, personal, and artistic needs into harmony with one another will determine your grasp of this aphorism's secret.

APHORISM NUMBER 33

**When you are not playing your instrument
Go about your day and
Identify yourself as being one with the Absolute.
Rest within a state of quiescence.
Thus rested and stilled,
Allow God's light and love
To flow through you.
Extend optimism, peace, bliss, and joy.
Help others as you find them.
Allow life to unfold before you
Of its own accord and in its own way.
Treat everyone and everything
As not more or less important
Than every other person or thing.**

Mind: Patanjali provides us with a practical list of activities designed to eliminate impediments to Ishvara. These suggestions facilitate a perfect blending of the Seer's spirit with the constant flow of spirit all around him. More importantly, these activities provide a means of bringing the benefits of a private spiritual path into the public world.

Body: The last five lines of this aphorism ask us to experience our day-to-day life with mindfulness and equanimity. While this might seem a daunting task, infusing common activities with mindfulness and equanimity is within the reach of anyone. Performing even the most mundane of chores in this manner elevates it to the level of spiritual exercise. A mindful task is one that is performed in a deliberate and unhurried manner. Regard the task as a delicate procedure that requires your full attention. Make no judgment as to how the task will turn out, allow it to progress organically, and be completely content with the results. When you find yourself thinking about something other than the chore, smile and gently bring your attention back to it.

Hand:
• Yoga Asana Posture: Performing Surya Namaskar, or Sun Salutation, aligns your bodymind with the hidden wisdom of this aphorism. This asana generates a preternatural trust and comfort that supports you in everything that you do.

• Yoga Dhyana Meditation: Asana: **Standing Pose**; Mudra: **Prayer**; Chakra: **2nd Swadhisthana**; Visualize: **Upturned crescent shape or the color silver**; Mantram: **Vam**.

Heart: In order to grasp the whole heart of this aphorism, you must wholeheartedly dedicate yourself to the tasks it concretely enumerates. As you do, revel in this truth; the Absolute is everywhere. It was never born and will never die. It resides in you, right now. Your only job is to use the experience of your yoga or music, to feel joy.

APHORISM NUMBER 34

When you play your instrument,
Pause after each note,
Gently restrain your breathing and
Observe where the note goes.

Mind: A mystic musician must learn to play one note with all the love, force, and emotion that he can muster. Even though the full range of technique, composition, and theory are at his fingertips, the Seer must reduce it to the act of playing one note and one note only. Only then will his art resonate across time. For the one breath and the one note brings clarity that eliminates spiritual and emotional confusion. Neither the Yogi nor the musician should perform their art as a frivolous diversion. Rather, they should play for the spiritual welfare of all.

Body: Engaging in activities that are fundamentally nourishing will support the wisdom of this aphorism.

Hand:
• Yoga Asana Posture: Creating Anahata-asana or Heart Pose, supports this aphorism. It activates the energy of

community and belonging while fostering a sense of yourself as a member of the universal family.

- Yoga Dhyana Meditation: Asana: **Half-Lotus Pose or Stability Lotus Pose**; Mudra: **Prayer**; Chakra: **4th Anahata**; Visualize: **6-pointed star shape or the color light blue**; Mantram: **Yam**.

Heart: Take your place in the Universe and enjoy life. Develop the ability to look at the totality of the whole and see it in each small individual part. Here is where you will find the secret of this aphorism.

APHORISM NUMBER 35

**Delicately remove yourself
From the notes you play and
Observe the effects each one has on you.**

Mind: Metaphorically pull back awareness of yourself as if trying to observe from a distance. Your goal is to see the totality of the bodymind while being mindfully aware of the sensations it experiences. This is essentially the same skill mentioned in the previous aphorism.

Following a single note as it fades away to its source generates a brief moment of mental clarity. This clarity can then be cultivated and encouraged. Treating a physical sensation like a musical note and non-judgmentally observing it as it fades away will generate that very same clarity.

Body: Any activity that stimulates the intuition will support the wisdom of this aphorism.

Hand:
- Yoga Asana Posture: Salabha-asana, or Locust Pose, helps create the self-observation skill mentioned in this aphorism.

- Yoga Dhyana Meditation: Asana: **Butterfly Pose**; Mudra: **One-finger**; Chakra: **6th Ajna**; Visualize: **Oval shape or the color blue-gray**; Mantram: **Aum**.

Heart: Understanding the whole heart of this aphorism depends on your ability to be emotionally open to your feelings. This does not mean giving in to wishful thinking or letting one's moods run rampant. Rather, it suggests an application of intuitive analysis to determine the truth of your feelings.

APHORISM NUMBER 36

When a note or expression blissfully moves you,
Stand before it in astonishment and wonder.
Watch it carefully;
See how it unfolds;
Make no conclusions about it.

Mind: From time to time within the phenomenal realm, each of us briefly glimpses the mystic quality of the world. If that brief glimpse can be cultivated and expanded, we can free ourselves from the tyranny of consensual experience. At that moment we become undone and released to our authenticity. For both mystic musician and yogi, this is the goal.

Body: Attempt to solve a problem in your life that you have previously regarded as unsolvable. Do not underestimate the difficulty you are likely to encounter. The energy released, as you move from problem to solution, will consolidate the soul and bring you into resonance with the wisdom of this aphorism.

Hand:
- Yoga Asana Posture: Bilik-asana, or Cat Pose, helps you see things with a renewed sense of wonder and astonishment. It also acknowledges our pranic commitment to and involvement with the world around us.

- Yoga Dhyana Meditation: Asana: **Chair Pose**; Mudra: **Vitality**; Chakra: **2nd Swadhisthana**; Visualize: **Upturned crescent shape or the color silver**; Mantram: **Vam**.

Heart: The secret to grasping the whole heart of this aphorism is the ability to relax and overcome both your physical and emotional tensions. True harmony resides in a successful reconciliation of opposites.

Things of great beauty possess magic.
Find something beautiful and
Without attachment,
Let it inspire your playing.
Observe how its wonders unfold before you.

Mind: Mystic musicians describe this experience as a marriage where flesh and music blend to become one. It is a hallmark of authentic playing. Staying non-attached to either the music or the beautiful inspiration for that music involves the Seer asking, "What do you have for me, today?" and being content and joyous about whatever occurs.

Body: Doing something to expand your horizons will put you in resonance with the wisdom of this aphorism.

Hand:

• Yoga Asana Posture: Ananta-vajra-asana (Eternal Thunderbolt Pose) fully integrates the inner and outer worlds of the Seer.

• Yoga Dhyana Meditation: Asana: **Kneeling Pose**; Mudra: **Cosmic Union**; Chakra: **2nd Swadhisthana**; Visualize: **Upturned crescent shape or the color silver**; Mantram: **Vam**.

Heart: Grasping the whole heart of this aphorism relies upon a quickness to act in the face of a transcendent glimpse of the world. Stopping to analyze what is occurring is a sign of attachment to the experience.

APHORISM NUMBER 38

Outline insights with your instrument.
Play dreams and fancies.
Pretend the Absolute and
Honor the Brahman with your Raga.

Mind: Finding passion and zeal within involves suspending the negative side of the ego. Too often, the yogi as well as the musician acts out of rebellion and approaches their art as a means of breaking ties with or casting something off. Unfortunately, in the process, we become inexorably bound to what we fight against and the negative ego dominates our being. We can suspend this process through musical improvisation. Expressing our nighttime dreams, waking desires, and intuitive insights regarding life itself.

Body: Walk with God as you go about your daily activities dedicating every thought, emotion and movement to Him.

Hand:

• Yoga Asana Posture: Virabhadra-asana I (Warrior Pose I) liberates the musician's spirit while fostering creative independence.

• Yoga Dhyana Meditation: Asana **Stability Lotus or Easy Pose**; Mudra: **Centering**; Chakra: **3rd Manipura**; Visualize: **Triangle shape or the color red**; Mantram: **Ram**.

Heart: The secret of this aphorism is resolute fearlessness and self-reliance. Harmonize your inner world and outer behavior towards your spiritual goals. Then, resolutely press forward.

APHORISM NUMBER 39

**Mystically join with an object
As you play Raga and
Uncover the secrets of the Pure and Silent Song
That lay hidden within the object.**

Mind: Mystic musicians, as a matter of course, routinely forsake outer consciousness and enter into deep union with trees, wind, rain, and other objects of contemplation. Thus joined, they musically express what they find. To discover the secrets of the rose, for example, you have but to play the rose.

Body: Throughout your day perform your activities as someone who has made a firm commitment to self-observation and investigation. Suggest to yourself that no matter where you go, every step you take is a purposeful step taken towards self-knowledge.

Hand:
- Yoga Asana Posture: Garuda-asana (Sitting Eagle Pose) generates an awe for the wonders of the universe. This awe is a vital component of the mystical joining mentioned in the aphorism.

- Yoga Dhyana Meditation: Asana: **Resting Pose, Butterfly Pose, or Easy Pose**; Mudra: **Prayer**; Chakra: **7th Sahasrara**; Visualize: **Unfolding lotus-flower shape or the colors of the rainbow**; Mantram: **Hum**.

Heart: The energy of the Pure and Silent Song constantly flows into every cell of our bodymind. It is the nourishing Brahman—the Absolute—in action. It is within this nourishment that you will find the whole heart of the aphorism.

APHORISM NUMBER 40

A Seer as a musician of the True Mind
Can play the whole heart
Of any object, emotion, or occurrence
No matter how large or small.
Truly, these things do not exist
Until the musician Seer expresses them in Raga.

Follow these steps
And the consciousness will begin to harmonize.
Soon thereafter,
The Pure and Silent Song will begin to manifest.

Mind: In the truest sense of the word, all music, and all asana strives to be poetry. Ubiquitous in the ancient world's mythic traditions is the belief that the poet is a maker who brings often disparate elements together to "make" an event in spacetime. Indeed, until the poet has expressed the event in verse the event itself isn't considered to be real. The Seer has the responsibility of preserving this method and using it to recreate the world whenever he plays.

Body: As you go about your day treat everything and everyone you come in contact with as a miracle. Allow these miracles to fill you with wonder and astonishment and you will resonate with the wisdom of this aphorism.

Hand:
- Yoga Asana Posture: Sav-asana (Corpse Pose) allows you to reconnect with your own innocence.

- Yoga Dhyana Meditation: Asana: **Chair Pose**; Mudra: **Silent**; Chakra: **1st Muladhara**; Visualize: **Square shape or the colors yellow and gold**; Mantram: **Lam**.

Heart: The key to understanding this aphorism rests in the ability to joyously celebrate all life events and occasions as they occur.

APHORISM NUMBER 41

**Harmonized consciousness
Produces the clarity and wholeness necessary
To still the surface of the pond.
As harmony builds in resonance,
Authenticity prevails and
The musician's True Mind
Begins to see what is before it.**

Mind: Metaphysically speaking, the important thing is not the ability to play the heart of any object or event. That ability is only useful because it facilitates the transcendental birth of the spiritual being within you. Harmony produces clarity, clarity stills the awareness, continued harmony expands the awareness, the authentic self is allowed to come forward, and the Seer begins to see with the True Mind. This is the virgin birth; the genesis of the mystic life.

Body: Living your day-to-day life in a free-flowing and flexible manner will build a firm foundation to support the wisdom of this aphorism. Intuitively move through your day and deal completely with the situations that confront you. Accept that forces much more powerful than your ego are at work within these situations.

Hand:
- Yoga Asana Posture: Ardha nav-asana (Half-Boat Pose) clears the inner vision, generating the clarity mentioned in the aphorism.

- Yoga Dhyana Meditation: Asana: **Easy Pose**; Mudra: **Balance**; Chakra: **3rd Manipura**; Visualize: **Triangle shape or the color red**; Mantram: **Ram**.

Heart: Recognize your own destiny and deliberately shape your life accordingly. Herein lies the secret of this aphorism.

APHORISM NUMBER 42

**This clarity and wholeness
Is the field of Tala, or rhythm,
Which must exist if we are to hear the Pure and Silent Song.
If there were no Tala
We would have no soul.**

**Words, ideas, and memories upon the field of rhythm
Can disturb the consciousness and give rise to thought.
But if the Seer behaves authentically
Within the musical moment,
Harmony will prevail.**

Mind: Behaving authentically in this context is often encapsulated by Gurus in the mystic music tradition with the use of the injunction, "Don't stop! Keep playing!" The field of clarity and wholeness has a momentum all its own and is expressed musically as Tala, or Cosmic Rhythm. If care is not taken, the fledgling mystic can get swept away by this momentum. This situation is remedied by tending to his musical creation, allowing it to "lean against the rhythm."

Body: Expand your sense of personal artistry and creativity to support the work and wisdom outlined in this aphorism. For example, if you have never painted, take up painting. Sculpt, carve, dance, or sing. Any activity that can be approached in a fresh and creative manner will suffice.

Hand:
• Yoga Asana Posture: Anja-neya-asana (Crescent Moon Pose) lays the foundation of spiritual insight necessary to maintaining authenticity.

• Yoga Dhyana Meditation: Asana **Butterfly Pose**; Mudra: **Prayer**; Chakra: **5th Vishuda**; Visualize: **Circle shape or the color white**; Mantram: **Ham**.

Heart: Plainly, the secret to grasping the heart of this aphorism is self-assurance. Proceed confidently as you move to encounter the infinite and abundant nature of your music.

APHORISM NUMBER 43

Resonance appears within the field of rhythm
And builds to a forward momentum.
Then, ideas, words, and memories dissolve
And move unerringly to their source.
When they have reached their source,
They return,
Giving rise to luminous musical expression.

Mind: Luminous expression, whether in music or asana, is not perfect and never should be. Perfection is an affront to God and a harbinger of spiritual ruin. Mystic musicians strive to play against the field of rhythm and are truly happy with whatever they produce. Indeed, they regard each and every sound they make as the most beautiful sound in the world.

Body: Perform tasks that you have absolutely no talent for whatsoever. Avoid becoming frustrated as you work your way through them and actively practice enjoying your ineptitude.

Hand:
- Yoga Asana Posture: Janu-sirsa-asana (Head-To-Knee Pose) helps generate a healthy fascination for the variety of life and experience.

- Yoga Dhyana Meditation: Asana: **Sitting Pose**; Mudra: **Balance**; Chakra: **3rd Manipura**; Visualize: **Triangle shape or the color red**; Mantram: **Ram**.

Heart: The key to understanding this aphorism is the ability to recognize when something must be broken off and discarded. This could be a habit, a professional project, or a personal relationship. Unbridled momentum can build to a frenzied pace. Know when to cut it off and you will have the key to luminous musical expression in the palm of your hand.

APHORISM NUMBER 44

Everything that is bathed in this luminosity
Opens up and reveals its whole heart
To both the player and the listener.

This is the music
That heralds the arrival of the Pure and Silent
Song.

Mind: To the mystic musician all objects are musical objects. In fact, all things are music. To experience that reality we have to educe or draw out the music from the core of the object by bathing it in luminous musical expression. As the educed music manifests in our awareness it begins to outline the Absolute and the Pure and Silent Song emerges from the space between the notes. Indeed, the Absolute becomes the space between the notes.

Body: During your daily activities, imagine that your motive force gathers to and issues forth from the lower abdomen. For example, when walking up a flight of stairs imagine that you are being pulled by an invisible rope tied around your lower abdomen. At the very least, endeavor to rest a portion of your awareness on the second or Swadhisthana Chakra as you go about your normal tasks and chores.

Hand:
- Yoga Asana Posture: Upavistha kona-asana (Seated Angle Pose) enhances the ability to connect intimately with people, objects ,and events. This intimate connection supports the eduction process mentioned in the commentary.

- Yoga Dhyana Meditation: Asana: **Sitting Pose**; Mudra: **Centering**; Chakra: **2nd Swadhisthana**; Visualize: **Upturned crescent shape or the color silver**; Mantram: **Vam**.

Heart: While it might seem counter-intuitive, the freedom necessary to luminous expression must, at this stage of the mystic process, be checked with stability and a sense of control. Establish clear emotional boundaries in all of your artistic endeavors and you will glimpse the secret of this aphorism.

APHORISM NUMBER 45

**The luminosity increases
As the Pure and Silent Song struggles to come forward.
It seems to emerge from within the player**

While, at the same time,
Seems to issue forth
From the very air around the player.

To the Musician as Seer
This is called the Formless Raga.

Mind: The situation described in this aphorism indicates a balancing of spiritual ideals with spiritual work. Indeed, Patanjali specifically tells us what this success at balancing looks like. It is also a picture of enharmonic resonance that progressively builds to involve more and more things within the musician's field of influence, which expands as well. The musician—now a complete Seer—becomes the immovable center within the consensual realm.

Body: At this point in the life of a mystic there is a tendency to become obsessed with fulfilling higher goals and ideals. It is at this juncture that the fledgling Seer is reminded by the Guru that he is not cultivating the path in order to fix anything or right some wrong. As a practical matter, it is important to learn when not to do something.

Hand:
• Yoga Asana Posture: Hala-asana (The Plough Pose) elevates overall levels of prana throughout the bodymind. It accomplishes this by absorbing terrestrial prana from the environment.

• Yoga Dhyana Meditation: Asana: **Kneeling Pose or Rishi Pose**; Mudra: **Cosmic Union**; Chakra: **1st**

Muladhara; Visualize: **Square shape or the colors yellow and gold**; Mantram: **Lam**.

Heart: If you can learn to differentiate between a healthy spiritual striving and obsession, then you will understand this aphorism and its importance in the grander scheme of things.

APHORISM NUMBER 46

Harmonized consciousness;
Clarity and wholeness;
Resonance and authenticity;
The field of *Tala* and
Luminosity.

These lie at the heart of existence.
The Seer as Musician
Brings them together in Raga.

Mind: The elements enumerated in this aphorism are those the mystic musician brings together to create the musical moment. Above all, this is a peaceful relationship of which the Seer is a full partner. These elements must come together in a spirit of reconciliation and compromise. If that cooperation is successful, the transcendental and innocent core of the Raga condenses. While the poet creates an event in spacetime with verse, the dynamic elements of the musical event, in this case, create the musician.

Body: Balance your day with equal amounts of work and leisure. If the first part of your day is cerebral make the second part physical. Seeking balance between contrasting opposites puts you in touch with the spirit of this aphorism.

Hand:
- Yoga Asana Posture: Bal-asana Child (or Infant Pose) reintroduces you to the doubt-free consciousness of a child at play.

- Yoga Dhyana Meditation: Asana: **Chair Pose**; Mudra: **Silent**; Chakra: **2nd Swadhisthana**; Visualize: **Upturned crescent shape or the color silver**; Mantram: **Vam**.

Heart: Whether you are creating yoga asana or music, remember that whatever you create should be regarded as a living thing and treated as such. Your mystic creation has come into existence for the sole purpose of catalyzing your spiritual well-being.

APHORISM NUMBER 47

**If he is successful in his musical expression
The True Mind gradually reveals itself and
He becomes the formlessness
Of the Pure and Silent Song.**

Mind: Patanjali plainly states that in the presence of lucidity and mystic awareness, the surface of the pond becomes still and reveals the Seer's original nature.

Body: Form an easy-going relationship with the demands of your day-to-day existence. Rather than focusing on specific tasks or positions, take a broader view and observe things from a healthy distance. Remaining flexible and objective will help you resonate with the message of this aphorism.

Hand:
- Yoga Asana Posture: Surya Namaskar (Sun Salutation) facilitates a perfect blending of spirit and prana. This blending supports the wisdom of the aphorism.

- Yoga Dhyana Meditation: Asana **Standing Pose**; Mudra: **Lotus**; Chakra: **4th Anahata**; Visualize: **6-pointed star shape or the color light blue**; Mantram: **Yam**.

Heart: There is absolutely nothing more important to the Seer than surrendering to authenticity. If you can accept the notion that you must play your own song and not someone else's, then you will begin to understand the heart of this aphorism.

APHORISM NUMBER 48

Great wisdom flows from the Pure and Silent Song.
It points straight to the heart.
It is universal, specific, subtle, and grand.
It is music.

Mind: The mystic wisdom that arises from the Pure and Silent Song guides each of us on our own unique path. It speaks to us directly and addresses those issues that are relevant to our personal existence. What could be better?

Body: Spending time with friends but not clinging to them will help you to grasp the full meaning of this aphorism.

Hand:
- Yoga Asana Posture: Parsva-uttana-asana (Sideways Bend Pose) and the meditation that follows generates the spiritual ease necessary to fully understanding this aphorism.

- Yoga Dhyana Meditation: Asana: **Full Lotus Pose, Stability Lotus Pose, or Easy Pose**; Mudra: **One-finger**; Chakra: **4th Anahata**; Visualize: **6-pointed star shape or the color light blue**; Mantram: **Yam**.

Heart: The whole heart of this aphorism rests in the knowledge that great wisdom is also common wisdom.

APHORISM NUMBER 49

**Musical wisdom
Revealed through the way of Raga,
Is far superior
To any other wisdom or knowledge.**

**This is because it floats upon the Pure and Silent Song
And issues from the True Mind.**

Mind: The art of mystic musicianship exists in a world of form and energy. The balance of physical form and spiritual energy is easily destroyed by inflexible or lopsided expectations. To avoid this situation, superior wisdom accessed with music must be handled delicately. When, during the playing of Raga, cascades of wisdom descend upon the Seer he should avoid drawing any conclusions about it. Rather than speculating on the insights, the mystic musician simply flows with the experience. He trusts that in the future this wisdom will reappear to inform his behavior regarding a specific situation.

Body: Any activity that is fundamentally nourishing supports this message of this aphorism.

Hand:
• Yoga Asana Posture: Adho mukha svan-asana II (Downward-Facing Dog II) promotes the precise blending of physical form and spiritual energy necessary to comprehend the scope of musical wisdom.

• Yoga Dhyana Meditation: Asana: **Kneeling Pose**; Mudra: **Diamond**; Chakra: **7th Sahasrara**; Visualize: **Lotus-flower shape or the colors of the rainbow**; Mantram: **Hum**.

Heart: Overcoming internal contradictions is the key to grasping the heart of this aphorism. Being comfortable with oneself is absolutely essential to walking the mystic path.

APHORISM NUMBER 50

Musical wisdom that gently floats
Upon the Pure and Silent Song
Is composed of layers of subtle resonance
That can still the consciousness
So completely
That disturbances upon the surface of the pond
Simply
Cannot occur.

Mind: The music that a Seer plays fundamentally protects and nourishes the True Mind. This is true for both the musician as well as those attending the creation of the music. It is within the influence of art designed to comfort and nurture that individual authenticity can emerge.

Body: During your day, look around for situations that have remained unresolved for some time. Bring those individuals and elements together and peacefully work to come to a genuine solution. This kind of interpersonal behavior supports the wisdom of this aphorism.

Hand:
- Yoga Asana Posture: Surya Namaskar (Sun Salutation) reveals the layers of subtle resonance described in the aphorism.

- Yoga Dhyana Meditation: Asana: **Standing Pose**; Mudra: **Cosmic Union**; Chakra: **7th Sahasrara**; Visualize: **Lotus-flower shape or the colors of the rainbow**; Mantram: **Hum**.

Heart: Music that comes from the thinking mind is the worst kind of fiction. Rather, authentic music flows out of the feeling heart.

APHORISM NUMBER 51

**Eventually, even the layers of subtle resonance
And accompanying hidden vibrations
Fade to formlessness.
Then, the Pure and Silent Song manifests completely
And the True Mind of the Seer
Is completely revealed.**

Such is the power of music.

Mind: With this aphorism Patanjali describes the point at which the Seer experiences the totality of the self. That all illusion, pain, habit, confusion, obsession, and attachment can be eliminated through music is profound indeed.

Body: Rather than focusing on areas of lack in your life, revel in your inner wealth and learn to appreciate what you have already accomplished. As you become fully aware of the inner and outer abundance you already possess you will begin to resonate with the wisdom of the aphorism.

Hand:
- Yoga Asana Posture: Ardha nav-asana (Half-boat Pose) supports this aphorism by generating the ability to see through complicated ideas and situations.

- Yoga Dhyana Meditation: Asana: **Easy Pose**; Mudra: **Balance**; Chakra: **3rd Manipura**; Visualize: **Triangle shape or the color red**; Mantram: **Ram**.

Heart: The whole heart of this aphorism is simple and applies to the practice of yoga, music, and life; follow joy and move towards happiness.

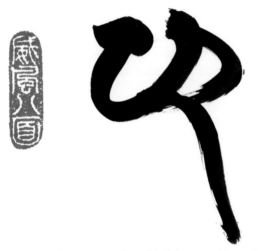

Paramartha / Ultimate Meaning

SUTRA BOOK 2

The Path to Realization
Sadhana Pada

The second Sutra deals with the practice of music as a
yogic activity. These are the actual training techniques of
the esoteric music tradition.

The Yoga of authentic music and
The music of authentic Yoga
Rests entirely
Upon only three building blocks.
All technique,
All method, and
All performance
Is evaluated against these three things.
Ask yourself these questions:
Is it the product of spontaneous discipline?
Is it the product of inspired and intuitive inquiry?
Is the entire self aligned towards Pure and Silent Song?

Mind: The strength of authentic music lies in its depth. It possesses infinite capacity to express life, absorb its essence, and support its movement. The very nature of authentic music—for this is a definition of authenticity—is one of balance and receptivity. The Seer must be open, docile, and nurturing while at the same time fiercely individualistic, willfully dedicated, and spirited enough to get through the inherent difficulties of the journey.

The music created along the way must conform to a very high standard if it is to be called mystical music. First, the study of the musician's craft must be unforced and completely uncontrived. The desire to learn the rules of the craft and how to apply them should never be regarded as a duty. Instead, the Seer becomes the obedient vessel where they reside. Secondly, all musical study and experimentation must be self-directed and intuitive in nature. The soul must come forward and lead the musician to the next note, question, concept, and creative idea. Thirdly, the totality of the musician's endeavors—from start to finish—must reflect a single-minded musical search for pure awareness.

Body: Make of yourself an empty canvas and allow the energies of your day to express themselves upon it. Rather than following a specific plan, intuitively feel your way along. Consider carefully where you go and with whom you meet. Patiently allow your wise inner self to tell you the best course of action and then take it.

Hand:
- Yoga Asana Posture: Bilik-asana (Cat or Kitten Pose) promotes deep feelings of stability and confidence while, at the same time, fostering vigorous curiosity.

- Yoga Dhyana Meditation: Asana: **Chair Pose**; Mudra: **Vitality**; Chakra: **2nd Swadhisthana**; Visualize: **Upturned crescent shape or the color silver**; Mantram: **Vam**.

Heart: Grasping the secret of this aphorism depends upon your ability to be patiently responsive to your life. If you can open up to the all-encompassing love of the musical journey without succumbing to starry-eyed fantasy, you will soon come upon the whole heart of Patanjali's message.

APHORISM NUMBER 2

**This is the music of
Complete union with the Absolute.
It subdues confusion,
Eliminates friction, and
Engenders wholeness.**

Mind: Authentic music is active, tenacious, and thoroughly dynamic. Amid the dynamism, the essence of existence is distilled—spun down to the fundamental sound of creation itself. This refined element cures suffering, thereby allowing us to fully integrate our being. This is the mystical musician's motive force for living.

Body: To align yourself with the wisdom of this aphorism, try something new today. Infuse your involvement with playfulness and complete impartiality.

Hand:
- Yoga Asana Posture: Parsva-uttana-asana (Sideways Bend Pose) generates a need to joyfully express oneself and supports that creativity.

- Yoga Dhyana Meditation: Asana **Full Lotus Pose, Stability Lotus Pose, or Easy Pose**; Mudra: **One-finger**; Chakra: **4th Anahata**; Visualize: **A 6-pointed star shape or the color light blue**; Mantram: **Yam**.

Heart: The whole heart of this aphorism can be found within your ability to know precisely when Heaven wants to speak and work through you. This requires a permission granted to the self to remain opened and poised. Only then will you receive its power.

APHORISM NUMBER 3

**Music eliminates the confusion, suffering, and friction
That comes from the habit of
Not seeing things in their true light.
It counters over-reliance on the senses.
It exposes the trap of consonance.
It subdues the winds of dissonance.
It eliminates attachment to life and living.**

Mind: In the previous Sutra, Patanjali outlines the main goal of Yoga practice, namely mystic union or Samadhi. In Sadhana Pada, he addresses the Yogic life and practice of the Seer in a more general way. Traditionally, Indian musicians have turned to this Sutra for advice on how to approach their life as an artist. It encourages the Seer to allow their attachment to mundane existence to come to an end and to embrace mysticism as a means of overcoming the material world. This is a quest for the truth of transcendental consciousness.

The mystic light of truth penetrates the shadows of ignorance. As a result, the Seer is introduced to the fallibility of the senses. As imperfect instruments, the sensory organs do their best. However, the habits and prejudices of the thinking mind distort and alter our perception, causing confusion and suffering. With the power of authentic music, this situation is remedied.

Body: Your perception of the world is just that—*your* perception. To align your daily behavior with the wisdom of this aphorism is to confront your own impermanence and accept your fallibility. Rely on your intuition to show your courses of action.

Hand:

- Yoga Asana Posture: Surya Namaskar (Sun Salutation) unites the energies of the sense organs and lays the proper foundation for a mystical understanding of this aphorism.

- Yoga Dhyana Meditation: Asama **Standing Pose**; Mudra: **Prayer**; Chakra: **2nd Swadhisthana**; Visualize: **Upturned crescent shape or the color silver**; Mantram: **Vam**.

Heart: Simply put, the secret of this aphorism is laughter. Laughter restores the senses, clears the lungs, and freshens the mind. When we laugh amidst a field of rambunctious joy we are, for a time, freed of our attachments. Laughter is a tool for breaching our habitual ways of thinking and perceiving the world around us.

APHORISM NUMBER 4

**Not seeing things in their true light
Sows the seeds of every kind of suffering
And gives nourishment to unwanted seeds already
sown.
It is the foundation of discontent.**

Mind: Not seeing things in their true light leads to all kinds of confusion and false perceptions. While the act of "looking but not seeing" causes full-blown delusion in the present, it also causes the undeveloped seeds of delusion from your past to grow. Mystics tell us that we are conscious of only of a small percentage of what we actually perceive from the outside world. Indeed, most of the signals we take in from our environment never make it to our conscious awareness. Instead, they are absorbed deep within our unconscious mind. These misperceptions of the distant past can blossom to full force in the present when we fail to see a thing in its true light. This can lead to feelings of depression without any apparent cause.

Body: Renewing contact with your own innocence will put you in alignment with this aphorism. However, being innocent does not mean that you should embrace naiveté or credulousness. Being innocent requires that you give up being and acting like an expert on life and living.

Hand:
• Yoga Asana Posture: Parvsa-kona-asana (Side-Angle Pose) condenses our spirit while fostering a sense that we are at one with the world.

- Yoga Dhyana Meditation: Asana: **Stability Lotus Pose or Easy Pose**; Mudra: **Centering**; Chakra: **3rd Manipura**; Visualize: **Triangle shape or the color red**; Mantram: **Ram**.

Heart: Previously sown seeds of discontent can cause waves of disruption that block the will. Stopping that disruption requires a clear and uncomplicated devotional life. Consistently follow your spiritual goals and don't allow inevitable disappointments and obstructions to put you off the path. If you can stay the course in the face of all manner of confusion then you will grasp the whole heart of this aphorism.

APHORISM NUMBER 5

**Without musically inspired intuition
You will not be able to see
Things in their true light.
You will confuse the authentic with the inauthentic.
All things must be expressed musically;
All things must be expressed yogically
If you are to see them in their true light.**

Mind: Intuition is indispensable to the life of a mystic. It is the heartfelt language of the soul expressed as insight, feeling, and emotion. It virtually requires feeling. Unfortunately, many approach yoga and music as a means of shutting off the world of feeling and emotion or, worse still, to be mindless. The way of the mystic musician, on the other hand, is to play an aspect of life as a means of seeing into it. The aspect of life becomes the inspiration and driving force for the music. Whether creating an asana or Raga, you are really converting yourself into a specialized light and lens specifically designed for observing life in its true light. But you will only be able to make this conversion if you take that same life as your source of inspiration and trust that everything will go well.

Body: Identifying with and seeking out deep relaxation will put you into alignment with the wisdom of this aphorism. Only when deeply relaxed will you regain contact with your intuition.

Hand:
• Yoga Asana Posture: Bal-asana (Child or Infant Pose) establishes a firm foundation for the wisdom expressed in this aphorism by inducing deep relaxation and building penetrating wonder and astonishment for the world around you.

• Yoga Dhyana Meditation: Asana: **Chair Pose**; Mudra: **Silent**; Chakra: **2nd Swadhisthana**; Visualize: **Upturned crescent shape or the color silver**; Mantram: **Vam**.

Heart: Trust is the whole heart of this aphorism. Specifically, this involves trusting the intuition when it speaks. Combined with deep relaxation, trust encourages a sense that your endeavors will evolve exactly as they should.

**But you cannot practice music's craft with your
senses
And you cannot listen to music with your senses
These are not things of the self;
They are things of the soul
And that is how they must be experienced.**

Mind: As a primary mode of being, authentic music is
not played with the hands, arms, and fingers. Likewise,
the ears only hear the surface sound of the musical notes.
The entire bodymind awash in a reflective state of poised
life force energy actually encounters the music and
allows the soul to interact with it. The soul, guided by
intuition, chooses which facets of the musical encounter
to emphasize and which ones to understate.

Body: Find some activity in your daily life that can be
soul-guided. A walk in the park, cleaning your house
mindfully, or intuitively re-arranging your workstation will
suffice.

Hand:
• Yoga Asana Posture: Nataraj-asana (Shiva Dance
Pose) is a powerful asana for the musician. It induces
prana to wrap around the skeletal structure and
uniformly absorb into the bones, thus fortifying the life
force. The entire bodymind then absorbs large amounts
of energy from the surrounding environment.

- Yoga Dhyana Meditation: Asana: **Rishi Pose, Resting Pose, Butterfly Pose, or Easy Pose**; Mudra: **Centering**; Mudra: **7th Sahasrara**; Visualize: **Lotus-flower shape or the colors of the rainbow**; Mantram: **Hum**.

Heart: Developing a gentle optimism for life and trusting that everything will go well puts you in touch with the heart of this aphorism. Like the meditation and asana from the previous section, it stabilizes the *prana* of the bodymind.

APHORISM NUMBER 7

**The trap of consonance is sprung
When you move towards what is pleasing.
Move towards consonance,
And you sing its song.**

Mind: The aphorism is plain enough. What attracts us is just as disturbing to the surface of the pond as what repels us. Consonance means "sounding together." Mystic musicians will play alone or gather as a small troupe. Likewise, small audiences of only two to three individuals is considered the best playing venue. The small audience is present to observe the mystic exploration of the musician and to be personally elevated by spiritual osmosis. Large audiences present a problem for mystically created music. If the musician's creation harmonically entrains a large group of spectators, he runs the risk of being pulled away from authenticity by the collective force of their unity. However uplifting it may be for those in attendance, their experience can overwhelm the musician, who becomes attached to their involvement.

Body: To align your behavior with this aphorism, do something to broaden your horizons. Mentally play with new and interesting thoughts.

Hand:
- Yoga Asana Posture: Bal-asana (Child or Infant Pose) provides a firm foundation for understanding the trap of consonance.

- Yoga Dhyana Meditation: Asana: **Chair Pose**; Mudra: **Silent**; Chakra: **2nd Swadhisthana**; Visualize: **Upturned crescent shape or the color silver**; Mantram: **Vam**.

Heart: Your ability to cope with the unfamiliar is the key to unlocking the heart of this aphorism. The birth of the mystical being within you is the adventurous birth of your spiritual life. It is a journey in every sense of the word.

APHORISM NUMBER 8

**The trap of dissonance is sprung
When you move away from what is unpleasant.
Move away from dissonance,
And you sing its song.**

Mind: What holds true for consonance also applies to dissonance. Determining precisely what constitutes dissonant sound is largely a question of musical taste, style, and setting. Within the context of mystic music, however, the trap of dissonance involves the energy of distance. While the trap of consonance involves sounds and emotions that are in close proximity, dissonant sound pushes energy and emotion back and forth to widely varying extremes. In the hands of a skillful musician, managing these extremes can be very appealing. But they sacrifice a spiritual continuity that disturbs the inner attention necessary for walking the mystic path. That having been said, while dissonance can cause us to miss much of the hidden side of life, if it is used judiciously it ceases to become a trap and becomes a tool for clearing perception.

Body: In all of your endeavors proceed with caution. Be patient with those you come in contact with and let time work for you. Moderation in all things is the key to living your day-to-day life in accord with the wisdom of this aphorism.

Hand:
- Yoga Asana Posture: Adho mukha svan-asana (Downward-Facing Dog) is designed to focus the inner attention that is disturbed by normal activity. It also clarifies the perception necessary to see things hidden from normal sight.

- Yoga Dhyana Meditation: Asana: **Chair Pose**; Mudra: **Vitality**; Chakra: **2nd Swadhisthana**; Visualize: **Upturned crescent shape or the color silver**; Mantram: **Vam**.

Heart: Can you allow time to work for you? Spiritual growth, like physical growth, is a natural process that should never be rushed. If you can passionately encounter life without giving in to the temptation of reckless behavior then you will be on your way to understanding the concept of dissonance within this aphorism.

APHORISM NUMBER 9

Interacting with life in this way
Is a natural occurrence
That bedevils
Even the most intuitive and capable among us.

Mind: The traps of consonance and dissonance are an inevitable consequence of being human. As such, we must all deal with them. But it is how we deal with them that determines the depth of our spiritual character. Achieving and maintaining spiritual harmony while avoiding extremes of feelings, emotion, and behavior can be a daunting task. To the Seer, even the simplest of things are important tests of character. The mystic way to pass these tests is to maintain unwavering focus on spiritual goals. This firm inner resolve defines the character of the mystic musician.

Body: Be as creative as you are able during your normal activities. This will bring you into alignment with the wisdom of the aphorism.

Hand:
- Yoga Asana Posture: Parvsa-kona-asana (Side-Angle Pose) brings your bodymind into complete accord with the spiritual essence of this aphorism. Namely, it reinforces your spiritual unity with the world around you.

- Yoga Dhyana Meditation: Asana: **Stability Lotus Pose or Easy Pose**; Mudra: **Centering**; Chakra: **3rd Manipura**; Visualize: **Triangle shape or the color red**; Mantram: **Ram**.

Heart: Uncovering the whole heart of this aphorism depends upon your ability to overcome contradictions and apparent difficulties. Resolutely resolve the inner tensions that you normally carry around and you will find the strength to eliminate impediments to the mystic way of life.

APHORISM NUMBER 10

**But the wise and subtle musician
Learns to experience consonance and dissonance
While in their astral form.
In this way, the musician is able to see
The root of any problem.**

Mind: Within the Indian tradition, projecting the astral self is a fundamental skill of the mystic musician. Frequently this projection occurs spontaneously during the creation of Raga. However, a spontaneous projection is not as stable as one that is deliberately cultivated.

Body: A good working environment, successful business dealings, sufficient rest and an optimistic outlook on life support the projection of the astral body. Extending compassion and gratitude also set the stage for success in the mystic skill of astral projection.

Hand: As a preliminary exercise the Seer imagines that he is projecting his spirit out of the bodymind and into the vast universe. This point of projection is either the Ajna or Sahasrara Chakra. Once projected, he imagines that his spirit expands to encompass not only the imaginary universe but also the musical situation he finds himself in. Then, after several moments, the musician asks the energy of the situation and the cosmos to flow into his bodymind. Maintaining as much stillness and tranquility as possible, the Seer envisions the musical situation existing within a field of eternity and patiently observes the situation as it unfolds. With practice, the musician becomes aware of the life force energy shifting and moving within his bodymind. The musician uses his instrument to convert these subtle physical movements to musical expression. With practice, this exercise sensitizes the Seer to the specific movement of *prana* in the bodymind that gives rise to the projection of the astral body.

- Yoga Asana Posture: Sarva-anga-asana (Shoulderstand) boosts intuition to profound levels. It also engenders intimate contact with the Absolute Brahman.

- Yoga Dhyana Meditation: Asana: **Kneeling Pose**; Mudra: **Cosmic Union**; Chakra: **1st Muladhara**; Visualize: **Square shape or the colors yellow and gold**; Mantram: **Lam**.

Taken together, the preliminary exercise, the asana and the meditation balance the prana of the bodymind and are specifically designed to promote the controlled projection of the astral body.

Heart: Look to the wonders of nature for the secret of this aphorism. Walk in the park, enjoy the flowers, and consider the many gifts that nature bestows on us. Only then will you grasp the whole heart of Patanjali's words.

APHORISM NUMBER 11

Then, in their physical form,
They are able to perceive
Those shapes upon the consciousness
Caused by clinging to pleasure or displeasure.
They harmonize those shapes by mystically joining
With the moment.
This is the way of music;
This is the way of Yoga.

Mind: Within a musical context, the astral plane is where the essence of music coalesces to become something that can be experienced in consensual reality. Music, however, isn't the only thing that comes together on the astral. The essence of everything we can experience comes together on the astral plane. The astral body is able to traverse this gulf between the realm of consciousness and the physical world. The Seer uses the astral plane as a mystic vantage point from which to observe the way that consciousness—

and ultimately, our experience of reality—is shaped by our habits, memories, and attachments. This provides the Seer with the specialized knowledge necessary to begin the process of harmonizing the totality of the experience.

Body: Mystics experience the astral plane not as an unlimited expanse but, rather as a delimited field in which the consciousness is excited to a high level. Said another way, it is a box in which the moving energy of consciousness rattles around and builds its strength. When this strength reaches a sufficient magnitude, it breaks out of the box and manifests as something physical. Limits yield intensity.

To bring your life in accord with this aphorism, place yourself in a situation that calls for you to be resourceful and creative within delimited confines. If you are a landscape painter, for example, who typically paints on large canvases, choose to work on a much smaller one. Better still, don't use a canvas at all. Paint on a fencepost, a door or even a ceiling with the same attention to craft and detail you would give a large canvas. If you are a jazz musician, challenge yourself to improvise within the confines of a folk melody. Whatever you choose to do, challenge yourself to move beyond your comfort zone, create within limits, and you will begin to resonate with the wisdom of this aphorism.

Hand:
• Yoga Asana Posture: Adho mukha svan-asana (Downward-Facing Dog) builds skill at the inward focusing of attention necessary to maintain lucidity on the astral plane.

- Yoga Dhyana Meditation: Asana: **Chair Pose**;
  Mudra: **Vitality**; Chakra: **2nd Swadhisthana**;
  Visualize: **Upturned crescent shape or the color
  silver**; Mantram: **Vam**.

Heart: The secret to understanding the whole heart of
this aphorism is this: Practice does not make perfect.
Practice is perfect to begin with. This applies to music,
painting, Hatha Yoga, or anything that we as humans
can do. To the mystic, life is not a trial performance. It is
the main event and should be played that way.

APHORISM NUMBER 12

**The lingering and vibrating sounds
Of consonance and dissonance
Reverberate deeply throughout the bodymind
Causing finespun changes in the very fabric of
being.
These changes give rise to intent and manifestation
That can appear at any time or place in existence.**

Mind: The psychic movement and pranic energy of all
experience and action continues to influence the bodymind
long after the specific event has occurred. This influence
gradually changes us on every level. It shapes our
emotions and intellect. It even changes our physical body.
These changes, manifesting subtly or dramatically, alter the
course of our lives to the point where we become reactive
beings with, in mystic terms, no will of our own.

Body: Willfully choosing what you think about will put you in alignment with the wisdom of this aphorism. Rather than allowing what you think about to be chosen by what others do or say, believe or behave, deliberately decide what kind of thoughts you will think about.

Hand:
- Yoga Asana Posture: Surya Namaskar (Sun Salutation) and the following meditation awaken the inner vision to the dimension of creative intent that is the astral realm. With this awakening comes the revelation that we embody what we receive into our beings.

- Yoga Dhyana Meditation: Asana: **Standing Pose**; Mudra: **Cosmic Union**; Chakra: **7th Sahasrara**; Visualize: **Lotus-flower shape or the colors of the rainbow**; Mantram: **Hum**.

Heart: The secret of this aphorism lies in your ability to intentionally disperse and diffuse negative thoughts with positive ones. This is the transformative power of creation.

APHORISM NUMBER 13

**When the lingering and vibrating sounds
Of consonance and dissonance
Reverberate,
They become the wellspring and origin
Of birth, growth, maturation, and death.
In fact, every event and occurrence in our lives
Comes from them.**

Mind: Patanjali's words are clear. The psychic patterns of what we are habitually drawn to or repulsed by form the basis of our evolving existence. In essence, we are intimately involved in a self-sustaining process of drawing premature conclusions about our unfolding life. This is generally accepted by explorers of the inner dimension. What is, however, frequently missed by many is precisely how much power mysticism has to overcome these habitual patterns of thought.

Body: In order to align yourself with the wisdom of this aphorism, seize the opportunity to open yourself to new perceptions. Additionally, you should immediately act upon those new perceptions without any prevarication or second-guessing.

Hand:
- Yoga Asana Posture: Parvsa-kona-asana (Side-Angle Pose) is designed to promote a quickening of spiritual devotion. It rapidly consolidates the energy of your higher ideals and renews their importance to you. This provides a solid foundation for understanding the wisdom of this aphorism.

- Yoga Dhyana Meditation: Asana: **Stability Lotus Pose or Easy Pose**; Mudra: **Centering**; Chakra: **3rd Manipura**; Visualize: **Triangle shape or the color red**; Mantram: **Ram**

Heart: Grasping the whole heart of this aphorism rests in your ability to avoid excessive rationalizations. Eschew cleverness and avoid venerating intellectual accomplishment. The secret key to this aphorism is "impulse."

APHORISM NUMBER 14

**In our lives we will manifest
Joy, bliss, and pleasure
Or sorrow, despair, and grief
According to the breadth and depth
Of these reverberations.**

Mind: The mystic must recognize that he is personally responsible for everything he experiences. This requires a rather solemn awareness of one's own gifts and deficits. Indeed, we harvest what we have sown. It therefore is incumbent on each of us to know precisely what is planted in the garden of our being. The following aphorisms will continue to explain this process of mystic knowing.

Body: To bring yourself into vibrational harmony with your experience, you must deliberately reach for joy and happiness. During the day, when you are confronted with a negative thought, pause for a moment and offer one that makes you feel better. This will align your behavior with this aphorism.

Hand:
• Yoga Asana Posture: Nataraj-asana (Shiva Dance Pose) represents a dance of bliss and the powerful creation of the world.

• Yoga Dhyana Meditation: Asana: **Resting Pose, Butterfly Pose, or Easy Pose**; Mudra: **Centering**; Chakra: **7th Sahasrara**; Visualize: **Lotus-flower shape or the colors of the rainbow**; Mantram: **Hum**.

Heart: The secret to understanding the whole heart of this aphorism is your ability to maintain an inner balance. This hinges on employing just the right amount of self-observation and self-criticism, neither of which should dominate your personality.

APHORISM NUMBER 15

The authentic musician is insightful and open.
Riding upon the posture and shape of his music,
He is able to perceive suffering of all kinds
By rising above it.
Vibration and movement
Are attracted to
Vibration and movement.
The Seer knows that it enchants, as well.

Mind: The fourth line of this aphorism refers to "...rising above it." This has two meanings. First, it refers to the musician's act of entering the astral realm in a non-corporeal form. This is experienced as floating above events that occur on the physical plane. Secondly, it refers to an emotional distance that the musician maintains with the events as they occur. The Seer in the astral realm becomes a singularly passive observer of events as they transpire on the physical realm. Indeed, he may even be an integral part of the physical event. Yet, the authentic musician remains aloof to what transpires and, merely watches. He knows that Raga, songs, and music are never created; they are found. Furthermore, he knows that he will find it within this mystical region of essential experience. The subtle energies of the musician are drawn towards the vibrational commotion caused by physical events. These same energies become the vehicle of his inspiration.

Body: Throughout your day, do your best to avoid self-doubt and self-destructive worries. If you can yield to the force of unpleasant situations while maintaining a strong sense of self, then you will begin to understand this aphorism.

Hand:
• Yoga Asana Posture: Trikon-asana (Triangle Pose) helps reinforce the aloofness referred to in the aphorism. It also subdues the fear of being inexorably drawn towards the energies of an unfolding situation.

• Yoga Dhyana Meditation: Asana: **Rishi Pose, Half-Lotus Pose, or Stability Lotus Pose**; Mudra: **Prayer;** Chakra: **4th Anahata**; Visualize: **6-pointed star shape or the color light blue**; Mantram: **Yam**.

Heart: How you deal with fear and failure will reveal the key that unlocks the whole heart of this aphorism.

Yet, the power of music is this:
Suffering can be harmonized
Before it manifests.

Mind: Consider this for a moment: all anxiety, disease, pain, and suffering can be eliminated with music. When in the presence of an authentic Seer musically expressing the moment, current as well as future problems and fears simply vanish.

Body: Throughout your day consider how attached you have become to the unpleasant things in your life. For example, sufferers of chronic pain will often reject treatment that eliminate their pain because they have formed a kind of bond or relationship with it. Simply put, their pain has become part of them and they fear giving up a part of themselves. Discover those negative things that have become a part of your life and release them. This will bring you into alignment with the wisdom of this aphorism.

Hand:
- Yoga Asana Posture: Matsya-asana I (Fish Pose I) moves prana through the main energy pathways of the bodymind. These pathways are called Sushumna, Ida, and Pingala. When life force energy moves smoothly through these pathways, obsessive fear about the future is released.

- Yoga Dhyana Meditation: Asana: **Full Lotus Pose, Stability Lotus Pose, or Easy Pose**; Mudra:

One-finger; Chakra: **5th Vishuda**; Visualize: **Circle shape or the color white**; Mantram: **Ham**.

Heart: Music and the experience of being a musician has many facets. Many speak of being intoxicated by music or of being "in love" with music. But music is also a painful experience that requires the surrendering of the ego as a burnt offering to the relationship. Once you have grasped this idea you will understand the whole heart of the aphorism.

APHORISM NUMBER 17

How is this accomplished?
Suffering is harmonized
By exposing it to Anahad nada;
The Perfect and Unlimited Sound.

Mind: Unlimited sound is called anahad nada. It is the foundation and core of the Pure and Silent Song. Sometimes called the "sacred sound *Naam*" and the "sound of the abstract," anahad nada is the sound that emanates from the flute of Krishna. Shiva dances to its melody. It is the sound and the source of revelation to all mystics from all traditions throughout the ages.

Body: Anahad nada resonates all around us in a continuous symphony of grace. Ordinarily, though, we don't hear it because we are so focused on the activity of the consensual world. Yet, it is very important to humanity. Moses heard it on Mount Sinai as did Christ while wandering in the wilderness. The Buddha heard it under the Bodhi Tree and Muhammad in the cave of his awakening. Lao Tse initially became aware of it while listening to moving water, while Black Elk first heard it riding on the winds.

Throughout your day reflect on this vital unity among the world's great religious and philosophic traditions. As a more practical activity, rather than focusing on the differences between peoples, look for how we are all similar. Indeed, we are more alike than not. Cultivating an appreciation for these similarities will bring you into alignment with the wisdom of this aphorism.

Hand:
- Yoga Asana Posture: Adho mukha sav-asana (Downward-Facing Corpse Pose) introduces you to the world of silence where anahad nada resonates universal wholeness. In combination with the meditation that follows, this pose generates and supports a state of grace.

- Yoga Dhyana Meditation: Asana: **Chair Pose**; Mudra: **Silent**; Chakra: **1st Muladhara**; Visualize: **Square shape or the colors yellow and gold**; Mantram: **Lam**.

Heart: The secret power of anahad nada is concealed in its intoxicating innocence. To awaken to the whole heart of this aphorism is to awaken to your own innocence. Nurture yourself by seeking solitude and stillness. Balance the aspects of your inner life with the intoxicating innocence discovered in stillness and you will begin to understand the sound of the abstract.

APHORISM NUMBER 18

Bathed in the light of Perfect Sound,
The phenomenal world of our physical existence
Becomes our vehicle for liberation.
It shines, moves, and expands;
It creates wholeness and abundance;
It connects us to everyone and everything.
It is, at once, both sensual and spiritual.

Mind: To hear the Perfect Sound is to release the soul to function completely in the physical world. The soul takes the lead in your life and guides all of your actions and endeavors. The soul expands the consciousness to include an awareness of the fundamental unity of the entire world. It flows to all points of existence and phenomena. It uniformly carries us to the universe. This is a thoroughly joyous and inebriating experience. With it the mystic comes to regard the consensual world not as something that must be escaped. Rather, through the creation of music, it becomes his path, nourishment, and motive force to liberation.

Body: Learning how not to control life will put you in alignment with this aphorism. This requires elevated levels of trust in your own resourcefulness. Trusting in your innate ability to respond to whatever confronts you is a fundamental skill of both the Yogi and the mystic musician.

Hand:

- Yoga Asana Posture: Bodhi-asana *(Sacred Tree Pose)* and the meditation that follows, generates the ability to hear the Perfect Sound. Once you learn to hear anahad nada your perception will clear dramatically and give way to mystic sight.

- Yoga Dhyana Meditation: Asana: **Butterfly Pose**; Mudra: **Lotus**; Chakra: **6th Ajna**; Visualize: **Oval shape or the color blue-gray**; Mantram: **Aum**.

Heart: Your soul is the source of power for the complete unfoldment of the entire Universe. Herein lies the secret of the aphorism.

APHORISM NUMBER 19

**The sum total and complete truths of reality
Are, simply, the myriad manifestations
of the Universal Essence.**

Mind: The Universal Essence is comprised of the underlying characteristics of nature that make up reality as we know it. Within the tradition of mystic musicians, these characteristics are thought of as both constituent parts and stages of manifestation. First stage manifestation is experienced as objects that we can see, hear, and touch. The second stage is our experience of mind, memory, intuition, and subtle sensory perception. Stage three reflects the unconscious beginnings of thought and consciousness, while the fourth stage identifies the field of the undifferentiated and undefined power of nature. This natural power is present even before it reveals itself as manifestations on the consensual realm. All of the reality that appears before us exists in one of these stages.

Body: Aligning your behavior with this aphorism is simple: create something that you regard as beautiful. Allow the opinion of no one else to affect you as you seek to bring out the beauty in something.

Hand:

- Yoga Asana Posture: Garuda-asana (Sitting Eagle Pose) prepares the bodymind to maintain a continuous experience of Perfect Sound. In combination with the meditation that follows, it helps penetrate the illusion of birth and death that hides the Universal Essence from us.

- Yoga Dhyana Meditation: Asana: **Resting Pose, Butterfly Pose, or Easy Pose**; Mudra: **Prayer**; Chakra: **7th Sahasrara**; Visualize: **Lotus-flower shape or the colors of the rainbow**; Mantram: **Hum**.

Heart: The heart of this aphorism is sustained by the earthly power of sensuality. The stability of a committed relationship intensifies sensuality. The musician takes his art as one takes a lover. If you can take nature in the same way you will uncover the secret to understanding Patanjali's words.

APHORISM NUMBER 20

When the musician's soul comes forward and creates,
The Universal Essence is exposed
In the light of Perfect Sound.
Then, led by the soul,
The player as creator completely experiences
Both Sound and Essence
Within the phenomenal world
And expresses it as Raga.

Mind: The musician's life is a search for truth. By immersing himself in a mystic study of the hidden secrets and wisdom of sound he comes to know the hidden secrets and wisdom of the Universe. Past, present, and future manifestations in the world are laid bare before the creative musical expressions of a true Seer.

Body: Embrace an optimistic and upbeat attitude toward life and you will resonate harmoniously with this aphorism. Above all, have fun!

Hand:

• Yoga Asana Posture: Sukh-asana (Happy Pose) generates an innocent and joyful trust in the innate wisdom of the universe.

• Yoga Dhyana Meditation: Asana: **Easy Pose**; Mudra: **Vitality**; Chakra: **1st Muladhara**; Visualize: **Square shape or the colors yellow and gold**; Mantram: **Lam**.

Heart: The key to understanding this aphorism is recognizing that each of us shares a common divinity. In fact, holiness is the essence of every being. Grasp this and you will grasp the whole heart of the matter.

APHORISM NUMBER 21

**Music exists
To engender this liberating experience.
The physical world exists
To support the reality of the experience.
The phenomenal world exists
So that we might see ourselves within the experience.
What a joyful moment!**

Mind: Patanjali clearly explains the reasons for the existence of a mystic approach to music within the phenomenal world. Namely, to remind us of our divine connection to the absolute, to provide a means of realizing and nurturing that connection, and to provide a means of sharing that nourishment with others. Indeed, through his craft, the mystic musician literally becomes the creative force in a natural world that exists solely to preserve the truth of pure awareness.

Body: If you want to bring the spirit of this aphorism into your life then it's time to become a pathfinder. A pathfinder is one who enters the woods at the darkest

point and blazes a trail for others to follow. This will take
initiative and decisive thinking on your part as well as a
willingness to take risks. Start a new business project or
become self-employed. Begin a new personal
relationship or revive an old one with a fresh approach.
Anything you can do to embrace the opportunity for
growth will help you resonate with Patanjali's words.

Hand:

- Yoga Asana Posture: Paschimott-asana (Western Side
  Pose or Forward Bend Pose) produces deep feelings of
  profound comfort that is often described as "resting in
  the womb of the world." Clearly, this sensation
  supports the message of the aphorism.

- Yoga Dhyana Meditation: Asana: **Sitting Pose**;
  Mudra: **Balance**; Chakra: **2nd Swadhisthana**;
  Visualize: **Upturned crescent shape or the color
  silver**; Mantram: **Vam**.

Heart: Real growth is not an easy process. Yet it is
only through growth that we can truly "rest within the
womb of the world." The key to a complete
understanding of this aphorism rests with how well you
are able to embrace the transformative power of
revolution. Can you give up the old and replace it with
the new? If you can release your grip on what you
have been clinging to then you will step towards
eternity and seize the heart of the Patanjali's axiom.

APHORISM NUMBER 22

From this moment on,
The world will look different to you.
You will hear it as Sound and Essence;
You will see it as play and creation;
You will feel it as vibration and movement.
Consensual awareness will fade;
Transcendental awareness will focus.

Mind: Patanjali makes this promise to those who follow the mystic path of music: you will be granted insight into the eternal life cycle of becoming and being, potential and manifestation, and life and death. At this point, the consensual world appears to the Seer as a perpetual symphony in which he has a vital part. If he plays his part well, then he is granted a spiritual blessing of incomparable depth.

Body: Align your behavior with this aphorism by avoiding feelings of exhaustion and depression. Get sufficient rest and be on the lookout for oppressive circumstances. Even though depression is part of the human experience, it is important to address it immediately. Reach for that next good thought and play Pollyanna's glad game. Then you will resonate with the wisdom in this aphorism.

Hand:
- Yoga Asana Posture: Garuda-asana (Sitting Eagle Pose) lays a firm foundation for understanding this aphorism by penetrating the illusion of birth and death.

• Yoga Dhyana Meditation: Asana: **Resting Pose, Butterfly Pose, or Easy Pose**; Mudra: **Prayer**; Chakra: **7th Sahasrara**; Visualize: **Lotus-flower shape or the colors of the rainbow**; Mantram: **Hum**.

Heart: The degree to which you can be open to change will determine your ability to grasp the whole heart of this aphorism. Remember, in order to thrive, we must find the fortitude to keep growing even in the face of transcendent spiritual accomplishment.

APHORISM NUMBER 23

**The contrast of
Transcendental and consensual awareness
Will delude you into thinking
That they are inexorably linked
But they are not.
This contrast is useful
Because it reveals
The nature and nuance of each state.**

Mind: Some think that consensual reality is a lesser state from which we must escape. Furthermore, they believe that things in the phenomenal world are fundamentally corrupt and should be avoided whenever possible. Transcendental awareness, they feel, is far superior. This is incorrect. The truth is that if we did not have the consensual realm we would never come to know our true nature. Neither would we be able to understand the breadth and depth of our divine power. The fact is, we need them both to sustain our spiritual path.

Body: Throughout your day focus your will upon your higher spiritual goals. Being courageous and decisive will align your behavior with the wisdom of this aphorism. But above all, give up the need to be conclusively right. Remember, you are in a perpetual state of evolving ignorance and understanding.

Hand:
• Yoga Asana Posture: Vrksa-asana (Tree Pose) supports the wisdom of this aphorism by eliminating conceit, greed, intolerance, and egoism.

• Yoga Dhyana Meditation: Asana: **Butterfly Pose**; Mudra: **Lotus**; Chakra: **7th Sahasrara**; Visualize: **Lotus-flower shape or the colors of the rainbow**; Mantram: **Hum**.

Heart: The whole heart of this aphorism can be summed up this way; be ordinary and happy. That is precisely why the consensual realm exists.

APHORISM NUMBER 24

**At first, the Seer accepts this unity
Because the he has previously been cut off
From the Perfect Sound and the True Mind**

And does not yet understand
The nature of phenomenal convergence.

Mind: Patanjali tells us that the false unity of the phenomenal with the transcendental happens because, essentially, we aren't used to looking at the world with a mystic's eyes.

Body: You can practice looking at the world with mystical vision. For example, see the space between the bars as holding the tiger and not the bars themselves. Regard the periods of silence between musical note as being the real music. Listen to what people don't say rather than the words they speak. And as you listen to them speaking focus upon the spaces of silence between their words.

Hand:
• Yoga Asana Posture: Utkat-asana (Mighty Pose) unifies the life force of the entire bodymind and directs it to release the ego's suffocating hold on the spirit. This is a pre-requisite to the development of mystic sight.

• Yoga Dhyana Meditation: Asana: **Stability Lotus Pose or Easy Pose**; Mudra: **Centering**; Chakra: **3rd Manipura**; Visualize: **Triangle shape or the color red**; Mantram: **Ram**.

Heart: The secret key to unlocking this aphorism rests in the ability to allow oneself to be captured by the mystical life. This is the most important step one can take to insure spiritual development.

However, through his music
The Seer establishes his authenticity,
Reveals his essential nature, and
Becomes a Musician of the True Mind.
Then, the apparent unity
Of awareness and phenomenon
Melts away.
Indeed, the transcendental is unsullied
By the consensual and phenomenal.

Mind: Through authentic musical expression the Seer learns how to consistently see the world in a new way—with the eyes of a mystic. This new way of seeing eliminates the illusion of consensual and transcendental unity born out of contrasting and choosing. Said another way, the musician clears his vision by playing his music and subsequently sees the complete wonders of both worlds.

Body: Isolate a situation in your life that is a dead-end. Perhaps you feel powerlessness regarding your profession or are in a situation that is tearing you in two directions. Once you have selected your dilemma, simply "change your ways" and you will begin to resonate with the wisdom of this aphorism.

Hand:
• Yoga Asana Posture: Parsva-uttana-asana (Sideways Bend Pose) fosters the spiritual ease and calm necessary to nourish the mystic sight Patanjali alludes to in this aphorism.

- Yoga Dhyana Meditation: Asana: **Full Lotus Pose, Stability Lotus Pose, or Easy Pose**; Mudra: **One-finger**; Chakra: **4th Anahata**; Visualize: **6-pointed star shape or the color light blue**; Mantram: **Yam**.

Heart: At times, we each find ourselves crucified between the apparent contradictions of our world. The only thing we can do is change the way we look at things. If you are not willing or able to open up to this change, you will never grasp the whole heart of this aphorism.

APHORISM NUMBER 26

**If you express phenomenon musically
While being intuitively guided by mystic sense,
You will naturally separate
The original eternal essence of a thing
From its many changing forms.**

Mind: The implications of this aphorism are staggering. Phenomena are events in spacetime. An object such as a flower, rock, or a car is a spacetime event. So is a waterfall, a wedding, or the sorrow that arises from loneliness. All events in spacetime have aspects that are changeless and aspects that are constantly shifting and changing. When the Seer musically expresses an event he is able to separate the impermanent aspects from the permanent ones and experience the truth of phenomena. For example, when trees are harvested and stones quarried to build a house they are changed. In a sense, they die in order to give birth to the house. When a Seer mystically expresses the event of the new house, the changeless nature of the trees and the stone are revealed. The mythic power of forest and earth come forward. The timeless history of season, natural disaster, wind, and rain are contained within the materials forming the structure of the house. The Seer draws them out with song. Even memories of those who, in ages past, rested beneath the boughs of the tree are revealed by the mystic music. But even this is not the goal as Patanjali will explain in the next aphorism.

Body: When a mystic musician separates the permanent from the impermanent with musical expression, he is actually restoring an event to its natural order. This requires great sensitivity and a measured use of mystic power. It is a delicate proceeding. Find an area in your life that seems hopelessly confused or cluttered and tenaciously set about clearing the clutter and restoring order to it. In this way, you will vibrate harmoniously with the wisdom of this aphorism.

Hand:
- Yoga Asana Posture: Sukh-asana (Happy Pose) generates a simple and joyful trust in the wisdom of the universe that is necessary to distinguish the permanent aspects of a thing from the impermanent.

- Yoga Dhyana Meditation: Asana: **Easy Pose**; Mudra: **Vitality**; Chakra: **1st Muladhara**; Visualize: **Square shape or the colors yellow and gold**; Mantram: **Lam**.

Heart: How can you ever be sad when you viscerally know that the essential nature of a person or thing can never die? Nothing in our lives is ever lost or attained, for that matter. We have but to mystically free-fall into the consensual world to see the heart of any event in spacetime. If you can understand this truth you will soon uncover the whole heart of Patanjali's aphorism.

APHORISM NUMBER 27

If you can rest completely
Upon the original eternal essence
Of anything that exists in the consensual realm,
Then the music of your very soul
Will manifest abundantly and wisdom will flow
From the world around you
To the world within you.
Then, all knowledge will be harmonized.

Mind: This is the reason for musical expression. It is important to note that a mystic's perspective does not differentiate between the self and the totality of existence. There is no wall separating the mystic from the world. Whatever he mystically explores, he becomes. The Seer is not content to dash about over the surface of phenomenal experience. He must dive into its very heart and, as a consequence, he dives into his own. To paraphrase Whitman, he becomes multitudes because multitudes reside within him. This is the mystic harmony of knowledge acquired in the search for truth.

Body: Engaging in worthwhile and compassionate pursuits for the benefit of others will put you into vibrational alignment with this aphorism.

Hand:
- Yoga Asana Posture: Virabhadra-asana II (Warrior Pose II) builds the confidence necessary to employ the wisdom of this aphorism. It also fosters the emergence of moral maturity that will sustain a lifelong search for truth.

- Yoga Dhyana Meditation: Asana: **Stability Lotus Pose or Easy Pose**; Mudra: **Centering**; Chakra: **3rd Manipura**; Visualize: **Triangle shape or the color red**; Mantram: **Ram**.

Heart: The secret to the whole heart of this aphorism is the search for deep meaning achieved through the contemplation of anahad nada. It is the folds of the Perfect Sound of the Absolute that you will uncover the spirit of Patanjali's message.

APHORISM NUMBER 28

**When the music of the soul manifests,
It refines and purifies.
When the music of the soul manifests,
It immediately presents transcendental wisdom.
When the music of the soul manifests,
It unerringly leads you**

To original eternal essence.
For this is the way of authentic music.

Mind: The music of a Seer blesses everyone and everything that it touches. His is the hand that consecrates with every note it creates. It is a healing hand or a voice that restores balance and washes away corruption. When the soul comes forward as music all things are set right.

Body: An alternate translation of this aphorism geared towards day-to-day behavior might look like this:

When the life of the soul manifests, / It cleanses and restores everything around it. / It advises our every thought, word and deed. / It unerringly leads us to the truth of ourselves. / For this is the way of the soul.

When you can establish an intimate relationship with your soul and allow it to inform every aspect of your life, you will be aligned with this aphorism.

Hand:
• Yoga Asana Posture: Marichy-asana (Sage Twist) has the power to remind you of your place amid spacetime by constantly reintroducing you to your own soul.

• Yoga Dhyana Meditation: Asana: **Resting Pose, Butterfly Pose, or Easy Pose**; Mudra: **Centering**; Chakra: **6th Ajna**; Visualize: **Oval shape or the color blue-gray**; Mantram: **Aum**.

Heart: Be true to your feelings. Listen to your inner voice and trust it. It is the voice of your soul. This is the heart of the aphorism.

APHORISM NUMBER 29

As musicians,
We join with existence by:
Harmoniously controlling our outward behavior,
Harmoniously controlling our inward behavior,
Intuitively guiding our physicality,
Balancing, shaping, and controlling our breathing,
Tuning our senses to our inner world,
Concentrating the faculties of our mind,
Engaging in meditation and
Mystically harmonizing our lives with musical expression.
In this way,
We learn to prevent alterations
Of the True Mind.

Mind: In this aphorism, Patanjali enumerates the *ashtanga* or "eight limbs" that make up the tree of music yoga. Within the tradition of mystic musicians, these limbs serve as devotional activities that motivate, support, and shape the spiritual life of the Seer. They are explained in more detail as the Sutra continues.

Body: In order to lead the life of a mystic, one must learn to follow the discipline of the mystic life. Many think that the mystic path is completely free and open and has no restrictions of any kind. Nothing could be further from the truth. Mystic methods were invented by individuals like Patanjali who wanted to share their profound experience of life with those who would come after them. They have already done the work. Jesus was a mystic, as was the Buddha, Lao Tse, and Black Elk. In their mystic methods we have the benefit of their successes and their failures. We have a record of their discoveries in the form of Sutras, Vedas, Upanishads, Gospels, and Enlightenment poetry. It is up to each of us to recreate their experience as much as we are able, to build on it, and to pass on our wisdom to the next generation in as clear a form as possible. This is the way of the true mystic preserved in the oral tradition.

Hand:
- Yoga Asana Posture: Matsya-asana (Fish Pose I) specifically supports the wisdom of this aphorism.

- Yoga Dhyana Meditation: Asana: **Full Lotus Pose, Stability Lotus Pose, or Easy Pose**; Mudra: **One-finger**; Chakra: **5th Vishuda**; Visualize: **Circle shape or the color white**; Mantram: **Ham**.

Heart: Grasping the secret of this aphorism takes trust in the good sense of the message and methods of the mystic path. Only your loyalty to it will produce the results described throughout the *Yoga Sutras* of *Patanjali*.

You control your outward behavior by:
Not bringing harm or injury
Speaking the truth
Not stealing
Embracing Chastity and
Subjugating greed and avarice.

Mind: Harmonious control refers to a balance of naturally occurring or authentic behavior. If you indiscriminately harm others, lie, take what doesn't belong to you, act in an excessively lustful manner, and live a life of selfish desire then you will never be able to live the life of a mystic. The surface of the pond will remain forever agitated. If, however, if you can naturally follow the injunctions in this aphorism you will bring a dynamic balance to your life that will support spiritual development.

Body: If you welcome your day and greet it with open arms, it will bring you many gifts. Don't take these gifts for granted. Remember, the consensual realm exists so that we might plumb the depths of our true selves.

Hand:
• Yoga Asana Posture: Danda-asana (Staff or Rod Pose) keeps you alert and aware to the workings of your own ego. It also helps maintain the balance of behavior mentioned in the aphorism. Seers in the mystic music tradition refer to Danda-asana as "The Great Equalizer."

- Yoga Dhyana Meditation: Asana: **Easy Pose**; Mudra: **Balance**; Chakra: **2nd Swadhisthana**; Visualize: **Upturned crescent shape or the color silver**; Mantram: **Vam**.

Heart: The secret to understanding the whole heart of this aphorism is the act of expressing gratitude and thankfulness for the many gifts of the consensual realm. Say, "Thank You!" to the world and you will understand.

APHORISM NUMBER 31

**These five should be thought of
As natural and harmonious occurrences
That go beyond
Time and space,
Birth and death,
Class and station,
Skill or age.
This is the Great Vow and musician's bedrock.
He must embrace them
Or his music will accomplish nothing;
The Pure and Silent Song will elude him.**

Mind: Patanjali emphasizes that the outward behavior detailed in the last aphorism must be part of our fundamental makeup. Behavior that is forced does not authentically reflect our true personality. No matter who we are or where we have come from this is the way we must govern our outer lives. Failure to do so will produce a spiritually barren life.

Body: Governing one's behavior can seem like a very complicated and daunting affair. But, it needn't be. In order to align your daily life with the wisdom of this aphorism (beyond the obvious), you must find your bliss and joy for living in a simple, carefree, and loving state. This, of course, must begin with deep love and respect for yourself.

Hand:
- Yoga Asana Posture: Ardha nav-asana (Half-Boat Pose or Lazy Back Stretch) clears the inner vision and facilitates an effortless understanding of complex situations. In this way Ardha nav-asana supports the wisdom of this aphorism.

- Yoga Dhyana Meditation: Asana: **Easy Pose**; Mudra: **Balance**; Chakra: **3rd Manipura**; Visualize: **Triangle shape or the color red**; Mantram: **Ram**.

Heart: If you can avoid behavior that is reckless or that wears you down either emotionally or physically, then you will grasp the whole heart of this aphorism.

APHORISM NUMBER 32

**You control your inward behavior by
The practice of physical refinement and radiance.
You control your inward behavior by
The cultivation of peace and contentment.
You control your inward behavior by
The rigorous and self-disciplined training of music.**

You control your inward behavior by
The soul-guided study of the self.
You control your inward behavior by
The dedication of your music to God.

Mind: Having discussed outward behavior, Patanjali addresses our inner world. Indeed, these divine rules remind us of all moral codes upon which a spiritual life is built. The first enjoins us to cultivate physical wellness and an optimistic countenance regarding our bodymind. The second asks us to actively generate peaceful and loving thoughts within our consciousness. This leads to overwhelming feelings of contentment that overflow to the life around us. A rigorous and self-imposed study of the craft of music leads to the kind of discipline needed to govern our psychic behavior. That the demanding study of the self through music be independently directed by the inner being is the fourth commandment. As a culmination of the preceding injunctions, Patanjali flatly states that the totality of your artistic life should be dedicated to the Almighty. This is a powerful message, indeed.

Body: The skill of maintaining stable relationships in your day-to-day life is vital to aligning your behavior with the wisdom of this aphorism. Likewise, you should be aware of your responsibilities as a mystic living in the consensual world. Never flaunt your perspective or use it to another's disadvantage. Be gentle with the world and you will learn to be gentle with yourself.

Hand:
• Yoga Asana Posture: Upavistha kona-asana (Seated

Angle Pose) generates the kind of deep passion for the musical life that is necessary to sustain it.

- Yoga Dhyana Meditation: Asana: **Sitting Pose**; Mudra: **Centering**; Chakra: **2nd Swadhisthana**; Visualize: **Upturned crescent shape or the color silver**; Mantram: **Vam**.

Heart: Can you enjoy what you have achieved even as you are achieving it? Or are you so busy striving to live a spiritual life that you miss the life you are living? If you can open up to the possibility of your true self in a sensible and mature manner, then you will be poised to seize the whole heart of this aphorism.

APHORISM NUMBER 33

Noxious thoughts
That are unhealthy and poisonous,
Can be easily harmonized
By cultivating
Healthy thoughts.

Mind: This aphorism requires little explanation. Interestingly enough, many people find the idea of willfully substituting a negative thought with a positive one as either too simple or too difficult! Mystics will reply that healthy thinking is just as trainable as unhealthy thinking. The degree to which the idea troubles you depends upon your connection to life. If you feel separate from people and the world around you then you will have difficulty cultivating healthy thinking. If, on the other hand, you feel a connection to the world around you, then a complete change from a bad mood to a good one is but one happy thought away. Now, you only have to think it.

Body: Adjust your behavior to foster a sense of connection to those individuals you encounter in your day-to-day life and you will begin to align yourself with the wisdom of this aphorism.

Hand:
• Yoga Asana Posture: Bhujang-asana (Cobra Pose) remedies the sense of separateness that often isolates us from the life and people we encounter in the world.

• Yoga Dhyana Meditation: Asana: **Easy Pose**; Mudra: **Vitality**; Chakra: **2nd Swadhisthana**; Visualize: **Upturned crescent shape or the color silver**; Mantram: **Vam**.

Heart: If you can confront old thought patterns and habits of behavior with a clear determination to change them for the better, then you will grasp the whole heart of this aphorism.

APHORISM NUMBER 34
Noxious thoughts expand with intent.
Intention can be shaped and controlled
With authentic and holy music.
Even silent approval

**Of the poisonous and unhealthy thoughts of others
Will lead to suffering.
Consequently, we must always choose thoughts
That are healthy and nourishing.**

Mind: This aphorism speaks to the damaging power of unhealthy thoughts. An unhealthy thought is one borne out of greed, lies, and mistaken impressions. They are angry and hurtful thoughts about others. They are disparaging thoughts about ourselves. The power in these thoughts comes from their intention to do harm which can fill up the conscious mind to the exclusion of all else. Intention can be small and produce only an annoyance or it can be large and give way to a hateful obsession.

Patanjali tells us that hateful negative thoughts can be controlled in the presence of mystically created music. He also tells us that unhealthy thoughts have a pernicious effect even if we aren't the ones doing the thinking. It is as if the act of having a negative thought broadcasts waves of ignorance and suffering to those around us. These waves can give rise to ignorance and suffering within those individuals that are in proximity to the original offender. Said another way, unwholesome thinking is contagious.

Body: In order to bring your behavior into alignment with this aphorism, observe the behavior and demeanor of people around you. If someone near you has a noxious thought regarding another person, object or situation, attempt to balance it out with an uplifting and healthy thought of your own.

Hand:

- Yoga Asana Posture: Marichy-asana (Sage Twist) organizes life energy in the bodymind that has become confused by noxious thinking.

- Yoga Dhyana Meditation: Asana: **Resting Pose, Butterfly Pose, or Easy Pose**; Mudra: **Centering**; Chakra: **6th Ajna**; Visualize: **Oval shape or the color blue-gray**; Mantram: **Aum**.

Heart: Consensual living constantly presents opportunities for unwholesome thinking. Mysticism and music can provide the immovable center necessary to weather these distractions. If you can stand completely still and radiate love in all directions for all things, then you will be able to grasp the whole heart of this aphorism.

APHORISM NUMBER 35

When the musician plays
From a place that brings no harm or injury,
He projects a rarified space
In which violence and coercion cannot exist.

Mind: When a mystic expresses himself musically he banishes all doubt and fear by becoming vulnerable to the moment of expression. He radiates a sacred precinct around himself and is able to expand it to include those in attendance. When the Seer plays, he is transformed and becomes living proof of the transcendent. He actually becomes a realized being possessed of mythic power. In the presence of such a being, all brutality, disorder, and violence of any kind, simply ceases to exist. This is the power of a musician following the mystic path of the Seer.

Body: Radiating a cheery optimism as you go about your day will not only bring you into alignment with the wisdom of the aphorism. It will also elevate your mood and the disposition of those around you.

Hand:
- Yoga Asana Posture: Nataraj-asana (Shiva Dance Pose) supports the wisdom of this aphorism. It, and the meditation that follows, provides the strength necessary to play from a place of no-harm and no-injury.

- Yoga Dhyana Meditation: Asana: **Resting Pose, Butterfly Pose, or Easy Pose**; Mudra: **Centering**; Chakra: **7th Sahasrara**; Visualize: **Lotus-flower shape or the colors of the rainbow**; Mantram: **Hum**.

Heart: The secret key to unlocking the heart of this aphorism rests in your willingness to let yourself be God's servant and become transparent to his grace. In this case, the call is to be productive regarding the radiant projection of love, compassion, and healthy thinking. Work in God's world and do God's work. That is the secret.

**When the musician plays
The truth of his own soul,
His whole life becomes
Authentic and uncontrived;
A wellspring of truthfulness.**

Mind: A Seer opens himself to the guidance of his own soul and, with human hand and human heart, toils innocently to produce something immortal. He excites the energies of creation that flow through him from the unmanifested realm and gives birth to sound that heals and motivates. He plays not the song of another because the force and fuel of his creation comes from the very fabric of his own being. The Seer fashions truthfulness that engenders yet more truthfulness from the world he finds himself in. This is the promise of music.

Body: In order to resonate with the wisdom of this aphorism it is important that you know how to "go your own way." Live your life in a way that suits you but be sure to live it with a quiet pride. Self-confidence is inspiring to others yet it must be original to them or it means nothing. Express your life in the way you express your music because truly, each is an extension of the other.

Hand:
• Yoga Asana Posture: Go-mukha-asana (Cow-faced Pose) puts confusion to rout and supports truthfulness in all areas of your life.

- Yoga Dhyana Meditation: Asana: **Half-Lotus Pose or Stability Lotus Pose**; Mudra: **Prayer**; Chakra: **4th Anahata**; Visualize: **6-pointed star shape or the color light blue**; Mantram: **Yam**.

Heart: The secret to understanding this aphorism is this: play your own song and not the song of another. This is the whole heart of the matter.

APHORISM NUMBER 37

**When the musician plays
Only the music that God gives him
And refuses to steal from others,
Riches of all kinds flow freely and
Are conferred upon him.**

Mind: Here is a story. Once an old man presented a young boy with a strange musical instrument made of wood, gut, and skin. With wide eyes the boy respectfully received the instrument even though he had absolutely no idea of what to do with it. Then the old man pointed at the instrument and said, "There's beautiful music in there. Music to move mountains, change the course of rivers, set fires, and heal sickness. But here's the most important thing. There is music hidden in there that will make people happy." The boy stared at the strange object and tried to comprehend the old man's words. Then the old man put his hand on the boy's shoulder, smiled and said, "Why don't you see if you can find that music?"

The boy searched day and night for the powerful music hidden deep inside the instrument. He beat, scratched, strummed, and plucked it to no avail. Finally, determined to play something on the instrument, the boy plucked out the bare bones of a popular melody. It was a great struggle but he succeeded. When he could play the song from memory, the young boy expected to be satisfied with his accomplishment. But he wasn't. The popular song didn't make him happy so he put the instrument down for the day and went to sleep.

Later that night, God appeared to him in a dream. The boy complained to God about not being able to find the music hidden inside the instrument. He also expressed disappointment at not finding satisfaction in learning the popular song. God smiled and said, "Well of course you're not satisfied. That's not your song. I let you struggle with it to show you how important it is to play your own song."

When he awoke the next morning, the boy felt refreshed and oddly relaxed. He decided to forego playing the popular melody and rededicated himself to searching for the powerful music hidden in his instrument. God watched the boy from Heaven and was so pleased that he sent His light and love to the struggling musician. At that instant the boy began playing the most beautiful music he'd ever heard. He was amazed by its power. It was so beautiful that he vowed to play it every day.

Years later, someone asked the boy, now a man, where he had learned such powerful and beautiful music. He replied, "Well, I learned the first song on my own. But then, God gave me the rest." He had learned that the beautiful music his grandfather had told him about wasn't in the instrument. It was really hidden inside himself. All it took was God's love to bring it out. This made the man, now a boy, very happy indeed.

This story not only sums up the aphorism, but encapsulates the life of a mystic musician as well.

Body: What is true for the music in the story is true for the rest of your life. Live your own life and don't copy the life of another. Your real life is inside of you. All you need is God's light and love to bring it out. If you can treat even a portion of your time on earth in this way, you will align your behavior with the wisdom of the aphorism.

Hand:
- Yoga Asana Posture: Danda-asana (Staff or Rod Pose) balances the energies of your inner and outer worlds. Thus poised, the wisdom, light, and love of God flows down into you from heaven.

- Yoga Dhayana Meditation: Asana: **Easy Pose**; Mudra: **Balance**; Chakra: **2nd Swadhisthana**; Visualize: **Upturned crescent shape or the color silver**; Mantram: **Vam**.

Heart: The whole heart of this aphorism resides in your ability to be patient with your spiritual endeavors. Things of great importance cannot be rushed. Even though we live in a world that celebrates the sensational and the fast, choose to live simply, slowly, and patiently. Only then will the power of the Brahman reveal your life to you.

APHORISM NUMBER 38

**When the musician
Embraces chastity and faithfulness,
His music becomes exuberant and vital
And he overflows with life force.**

Mind: Chastity and faithfulness is this context refers to being faithful to the path of mystic music and remaining unsullied by outside distractions. When your attention is drawn away from the path you experience a loss of essence or vitality which is the motive force for living a creative life. Think of a loss of vitality and essence as a broken promise that you have made to yourself. This broken promise can leave you feeling empty and adrift. However, if you can keep the promise of pursuing authentic music in spite of distractions, then you will experience a near endless supply of energy.

Body: The loss of vitality has physical ramifications. Lethargy, back pain, and general weakness are but a few of the consequences. However, this malady often manifests an obsessive need to seek the approval of others. This need has no place in the mystic lifestyle. To remedy this situation, take steps to nourish your bodymind. Traditionally, this involves spending time in nature as a means of recharging your batteries. With the act of reconnecting with the natural world you will bring yourself into alignment with the wisdom of the aphorism.

Hand:
- Yoga Asana Posture: Baka-asana (Crane Pose) is designed to deeply connect you to nature. It also eliminates the need for the approval of others.

- Yoga Dhyana Meditation: Asana **Full Lotus Pose, Stability Lotus Pose, or Easy Pose**; Mudra: **One-finger**; Chakra: **5th Vishuda**; Visualize: **Circle shape or the color white**; Mantram: **Ham**.

Heart: To confront the need for the approval of others is to encounter our dark side. In these shadows we discover an array of unconscious forces that we thought we had been rid of. We were mistaken, for the darkness remains. Embracing the chastity and faithfulness of the mystic path will bring light into this darkness and, in the process, expose the whole heart of this aphorism.

APHORISM NUMBER 39

**When the musician
Embraces generosity and eschews greed,
His music unlocks a vast storehouse
Of transcendental and consensual knowledge.**

Mind: One of the many gifts of a life dedicated to mystical music is access to a great invisible library containing the secrets of the Universe. This library contains information about people and occurrences that have been forgotten in the consensual realm. Knowledge concerning past lives and future existences is what Patanjali chooses to discuss in this aphorism. Once you have knowledge of your past lives, you will know the divine purpose of your existence. And when you know the path of your future incarnations, you will know how best to fulfill your destiny.

Body: Avoid greed in your daily life and you will vibrate harmoniously with this aphorism. Treat others with respect and be generous with your time and attention. Remember, if you want love, freely give love away.

Hand:
- Yoga Asana Posture: Garuda-asana (Sitting Eagle Pose) invigorates all seven Chakras, especially the ajna Chakra which is the Spiritual Eye of transcendental knowledge.

- Yoga Dhyana Meditation: Asana: **Resting Pose, Butterfly Pose, or Easy Pose**; Mudra: **Prayer**; Chakra: **7th Sahasrara**; Visualize: **Lotus-flower shape or the colors of the rainbow**; Mantram: **Hum**.

Heart: The key to unlocking this aphorism is time and how you think about it. If you think of time as a thief that steals your life bit by bit, then you will be shut out of eternity. On the other hand, if you treat time with respect and see it as a traveling companion, you will come to understand the true nature of generosity.

APHORISM NUMBER 40

**Through the practice of radiance
And physical refinement,
The musician is able to align himself
With Perfect Sound and the body becomes
His finely tuned instrument.
Anyone in his presence becomes harmonized.**

Mind: Patanjali continues discussing the methods of harmoniously controlling behavior. The practice of radiance and physical refinement can best be thought of as cultivating physical wellness and positive acceptance of the bodymind.

Wellness in this case is a sophisticated stance regarding how we interact with the essentials of life. What we eat, drink, do professionally, and how we spend our leisure time figures prominently into wellness. Some believe that it enjoins us to strictly regulate our diet, for example, and eat only certain kinds of food. But wellness has far less to do with what kinds of food we eat and much more to do with how we eat them. If we regard our food respectfully and strive to have a complete experience of eating, we will be contributing to our wellness. Whether eating, drinking, working, or engaging in leisure activities, offer everything you do as a prayer thanking God for the wonders of life and asking him for more understanding of those wonders. Physical wellness naturally follows.

Cultivating a positive acceptance of the bodymind is a natural extension of cultivating physical wellness. It can best be thought of as a personal radiance that comes from a joyful participation in the wonders of your corporeal self. Rather than thinking of yourself as a collection of disgusting parts that wear out and get sick, see yourself as a beautiful extension of the Absolute. Spiritual attainment simply cannot take place without a bodymind.

When a musician's life is informed by wellness and radiance, he becomes aligned with Perfect Sound. When his musical expression is informed by wellness and radiance, those in attendance become temporarily aligned with Perfect Sound. Thus aligned, they themselves experience elevated levels of personal wellness and radiance.

Body: Revel in your life; enjoy it deeply. If, at any given moment in spacetime, you can draw completely on your bodymind gifts, deficits, and assets and thoroughly enjoy that moment then your behavior will resonate with the wisdom of this aphorism.

Hand:
- Yoga Asana Posture: Marichy-asana (Sage Twist) unerringly reveals your place amid the flow of spacetime.

- Yoga Dhyana Meditation: Asana **Resting Pose, Butterfly Pose, or Easy Pose**; Mudra: **Centering**; Chakra: **6th Ajna**; Visualize: **Oval shape or the color blue-gray**; Mantram: **Aum**.

Heart: Regarding the bodymind as an unclean and disgusting thing reveals a fundamental misunderstanding of the mystic path to realization. Indeed, possessing a negative self-image is the cause of much human suffering in the world. While it is true that things on the consensual realm shift, change, and degrade, it is also true that the seed of decay gives birth to great abundance. Grasp this concept and you will be taken to the core of this aphorism.

APHORISM NUMBER 41

Radiance and refinement
Actualized in music
Brings the player composure,
Gladness,
Peace,
Adroit single-mindedness,
Dominion over sensual experience
Profound interior awareness.

Mind: Patanjali tells us what we receive when we bring wellness and positive acceptance of the bodymind to our creative musical expressions. Specifically, we experience abundant happiness, joy, and contentment coupled with overwhelming feelings of peacefulness. Expanded powers of concentration allow us to more thoroughly participate in our consensual life. Musically expressed wellness and radiance also grants us a near unlimited capacity to explore the depths of our inner world.

It is important to note that having dominion over sensual experience is not the act of exerting complete control over the senses. Rather, the Seer comes to understand his cooperative role with the sense as partners in creating experience.

Body: Clear-headed thinking and acting with self-reliant determination will bring your day-to-day behavior into alignment with the wisdom of this aphorism.

Hand:
- Yoga Asana Posture: Sav-asana (Corpse Pose) soothes the life force energy, allowing it to deeply nourish the bodymind. This ushers in feelings of profound peace and contentment.

- Yoga Dhyana Meditation: Asana: **Chair Pose**; Mudra: **Silent**; Chakra: **1st Muladhara**; Visualize: **Square shape or the colors yellow and gold**; Mantram: **Lam**.

Heart: The secret of this aphorism resides in your ability to attend to the minutia of life. Can you patiently and thoroughly take care of the small things? When you can remain calm and relaxed while attending to details, you will soon discover the whole heart of Patanjali's words.

APHORISM NUMBER 42

**Cultivating peace and contentment
And expressing it musically,
Brings blissfulness and great joy
To every part of the musician's life.**

Mind: When the Seer musically expresses the contentment found in wellness and radiance every earthly encounter becomes delightful. Events—even unpleasant ones—take happy and joyous turns.

Body: If you can behave as if everyone and everything you encounter in your daily life is, in reality, a part of or extension of yourself, then you will begin to resonate with the wisdom of this aphorism.

Hand:
- Yoga Asana Posture: Paripurma nav-asana (Longboat Pose), also known as Kriya-asana, induces a state of consciousness wherein everyone and everything you encounter is perceived to be a joyful reflection of yourself.

- Yoga Dhyana Meditation: Asana: **Easy Pose**; Mudra: **Balance**; Chakra: **3rd Manipura**; Visualize: **Triangle shape or the color red**; Mantram: **Ram**.

Heart: The whole heart of this aphorism is cooperation. The Seer cooperates with cosmic forces and is enriched. He also cooperates with the people he meets. The Seer brings his enrichment to the meeting which gives rise to enhanced perceptions for all those involved. These perceptions range from wondrous and surprising to validating and nourishing. And it all began because the Seer first cooperated with music.

APHORISM NUMBER 43

Rigorous and self-disciplined musical training
Purifies the body,
Perfects the mind,
Projects the soul, and
Fine-tunes the senses
To perceive wonders.

Mind: Walking the path of mystic musicianship is a fundamentally healing endeavor. It strengthens and heals the mind as well as the body. It allows the soul to come forward and lead us through a mystic exploration of the universe. Along the way, it transforms our awareness so we might see what it sees and, as a consequence of the transformation, be reminded of our own divinity.

Body: Throughout your day, do your best to turn your intentions into reality. While there is a time to consider things thoughtfully and make detailed plans, do your best to keep your eye on the prize. Remember, perfectionism is not the mystic's way. Be persistent and you will bring your behavior into alignment with this aphorism.

Hand:

- Yoga Asana Posture: Paripurma nav-asana or Kriya-asana (Longboat Pose) supports the wisdom of this aphorism.

- Yoga Dhyana Meditation: Asana: **Easy Pose**; Mudra: **Balance**; Chakra: **3rd Manipura**; Visualize: **Triangle shape or the color red**; Mantram: **Ram**.

Heart: When you are at peace your perspective is clear and options regarding your life look bright. And shouldn't they be? In the final analysis, every life is a work of art. This is the heart of the aphorism.

APHORISM NUMBER 44

Soul-guided study of the Self
Brings you closer to God.

Mind: Let me be as plain as I am able; an authentic study of the self through music must be guided by none other than your inner being. Any other course will be a cheaply bought compromise with your ideals.

Body: In all that you do, remember that your relationship to the Absolute hangs in the brink. Even the most mundane of daily chores can either bring you closer to God or push Him away. Confronting this reality requires a mindful awareness of the inner workings of your personality and how they inform your behavior.

Hand:
Yoga Asana Posture: Dhanura-asana (Bow Pose) universally stimulates the prana that runs through all of the subtle energy pathways of the bodymind.

Yoga Dhyana Meditation: Asana: **Butterfly Pose**; Mudra: **Centering**; Chakra: **5th Vishuda**; Visualize: **Circle shape or the color white**; Mantram: **Ham**.

Heart: Spiritual independence is the key to unlocking the meaning of this aphorism.

APHORISM NUMBER 45

**Harmonizing your life through music
Occurs when you dedicate your art to God
And rest upon the vibrations of Pure and Silent
Song.**

Mind: This aphorism is very clear. An alternate translation might be:

Bringing wholeness to your life with yoga
Occurs when you dedicate your practice of yoga to God
And rest upon the truth of pure awareness.

Body: Take comfort in the ordering structures of your life. If your daily life is unstructured, then it's time to impose order and be disciplined in maintaining it. If you are successful, you will come into alignment with the wisdom of this aphorism.

Hand:

Yoga Asana Posture: The Sasanka-asana I (Hare Pose I) when combined with the meditation that follows, provides the energetic balance necessary to support the wisdom of this aphorism.

Yoga Dhyanna Meditation: Asana: **Kneeling Pose**; Mudra: **Fire**; Chakra: **1st Muladhara**; Visualize:

Square shape or the colors yellow and gold;
Mantram: **Lam**.

Heart: When you can find luminous freedom within even the most ordered environment you will be able to grasp the whole heart of this aphorism.

APHORISM NUMBER 46

Your music should be meditation and
Your meditation should be music.
When you play,
Your posture should be
Rooted and comfortable.
When you play,
Your attitude should be
Open and Joyful.

Mind: Playing music—or listening to it for that matter—is the Seer's meditation. Patanjali provides us with sufficient instruction within the aphorism.

Body: In reality, it is desirable for the mystic to experience every part of his life as a meditation. Advice for this approach to life is, in essence, found throughout the *Yoga Sutras*. We have only to look for it.

Hand:
• Yoga Asana Posture: Surya Namaskar (Sun Salutation) supports the wisdom of this aphorism.

- Yoga Dhyana Meditation: Asana: **Standing Pose**;
  Mudra: **Cosmic Union**; Chakra: **7th Sahasrara**;
  Visualize: **Lotus-flower shape or the colors of
  the rainbow**; Mantram: **Hum**.

This meditation is also designed to be performed while
listening to music. It converts the comparatively simple
act of hearing into a profound meditation.

Heart: Through the practice of meditation we become
aware of the Absolute at work within the consensual
world. The more we become aware of the Absolute, the
deeper our meditative state becomes. The deeper our
meditative state becomes, the more we become aware of
the Absolute within the consensual. This is the whole
heart of this aphorism.

APHORISM NUMBER 47

**Then, you will be without exertion
And life force will flow unimpeded.
At that moment,
You will spontaneously identify with the infinite
And feel inseparable from it.**

Mind: Proceeding from the last aphorism, Patanjali
describes the awakening experience that occurs when
the Seer successfully plays his music as meditation. The
hallmarks of this experience are: 1) the Seer's bodymind
becomes a conduit for the free and unrestricted flow of
prana, 2) as a result of this free-flowing energy, the Seer

perceives himself to be an inseparable part of the boundless Universe, and 3) this feeling of indivisibility ushers in a fresh and previously unrealized state of profound relaxation.

Body: Within this tradition, the emergence of boundlessness is heralded within the substance of the player's dreams. The archetypes that appear in the dream state include images of a female warrior, stringed instruments, crescent moons, fruit, and flowers, among others.

Meditation provides the skills necessary for each of us to be aware of the substance of our dreams. In order to align your behavior with this aphorism, express to yourself the desire to remember your dreams. Keep a journal of the images you encounter or discuss them with like-minded friends. When you can easily remember the details of your dreams, you will be in alignment with the wisdom of this aphorism.

Hand:
- Yoga Asana Posture: Surya Namaskar (Sun Salutation) fully supports the wisdom of this aphorism and the experience of boundlessness achieved through meditative music.

- Yoga Dhyana Meditation: Asana **Standing Pose**; Mudra: **Cosmic Union**; Chakra: **7th Sahasrara**; Visualize: **Lotus-flower shape or the colors of the rainbow**; Mantram: **Hum**.

Heart: Effective meditation requires an abiding trust between you and your inner self. When you can unabashedly trust in the good sense of a regular regimen of meditation, you will be on your way to understanding the whole heart of this aphorism.

APHORISM NUMBER 48

Being fully relaxed, open, and joyful,
You will no longer be disturbed by contrast.

Mind: The Seer comes to understand the complete correctness of the contrasting Universe and its myriad manifestations within the consensual realm. This realization leaves the Seer joyful, radiant, and exquisitely happy.

Body: Throughout your day, contemplate the notion that everything in your life is precisely where it should be. Behave as if all occurrences in your life are overseen by a higher intelligence alive with causation. When you can behave as if everything in your world makes perfect sense just as it is, you will be in alignment with this aphorism.

Hand:
- Yoga Asana Posture: Ardha nav-asana (Half-Boat Pose or Lazy Back Stretch) clears the inner vision and generates the ability to think deeply into the workings of the contrasting universe. The meditation that follows accomplishes the very same thing.

- Yoga Dhyana Meditation: Asana: **Easy Pose**; Mudra: **Balance**; Chakra: **3rd Manipura**; Visualize: **Triangle shape or the color red**; Mantram: **Ram**.

Heart: The realization of the absolute correctness of the contrasting Universe should never give rise to the notion that we are powerless to affect it. To the contrary, understanding the contrasting Universe means confronting our power to radically change it for our benefit. Said another way, don't drift about aimlessly hoping for a miracle. Instead, make your own miracle. This is the whole heart of the aphorism.

APHORISM NUMBER 49

When your body is balanced and at ease
The breath becomes balanced and at ease.
The music played shapes the breath and
Eventually, the player,
Learning to control the breath altogether,
May stop and start it at will.

Mind: With these words, Patanjali establishes the art of *pranayama*, which means "to control the breath of life." Since that time pranayama has evolved into a complete field of yogic study. However, within the ancient tradition of mystic musicians, breath control is something that occurs spontaneously as the Seer's skill at music meditation grows. All of the wonders of breath control are revealed intuitively to the Seer who follows the mystic path.

Control of the breath is inexorably linked to controlling the life energy of the bodymind. Indeed, one cannot be had without the other. The Seer actually creates music that shapes the depth and quality of the breath. He can manipulate the inhalations and exhalations at will depending upon the way he chooses to express himself. As a result, he acquires great skill at manipulating the life energy with sound. He may even stop the breath altogether without suffering any ill effects.

Body: Set aside sufficient time to complete a typical daily task such as preparing a meal. As you prepare the meal, mindfully watch your breathing. Judge each inhalation and exhalation as being either rough or smooth. Divide your attention between the actions of meal preparation and judging the quality of your breathing. Soon, you will notice that you are moving slower and more deliberately. Your mental processes will be clear and comfortable. When this occurs you will be resonating harmoniously with the wisdom of this aphorism.

Hand:
- Yoga Asana Posture: Sukh-asana (Happy Pose) naturally regulates the breath. In this way, it helps support the wisdom of this aphorism.

- Yoga Dhyana Meditation: Asana: **Easy Pose**; Mudra: **Vitality**; Chakra: **1st Muladhara**; Visualize: **Square shape or the colors yellow and gold**; Mantram: **Lam**.

Heart: The history of Indian Music Masters abounds with stories of mystics who possessed superhuman powers as a result of learning how to control the breath. In some cases the populace even revered them as gods. But they were not gods. However, by intuitively learning the secrets of pranayama, I do believe they were touched by God. This is the whole heart of the aphorism.

APHORISM NUMBER 50

**The breath in all its permutations
Consists of inhalations, exhalations, and
Fixed moments in-between.
These three may be adjusted as to
Rhythmic beat, time, and rest
Until the breath expands from within
And becomes a subtle interior event.
Then, the surface of the pond
Will rest undisturbed.
Here, we glimpse the True Mind.**

Mind: As skill at intuitively controlling the breath builds, the Seer's relationship to it changes completely. He soon learns to match the rhythm and quality of his breath with the rhythm and quality of his music. Even the subtlest inflection of a note can affect the breath and vice versa. When during the course of his musical expression, the Seer finds a dynamic balance between the breath controlling the music and the music controlling the breath, he feels his interior ground of being expanding in all directions. It's as if the molecules of his bodymind uniformly fly apart to fill up the room. At this point, the breathing appears to stop altogether and inner disturbances that cause alterations of the True Mind cease. The Seer can then glimpse himself within the pond's pure reflective surface.

Body: Early in your day, make the decision to be mindfully aware of your breathing. As you go about your day, watch your breath and become aware of how different people and situations change it. Also be aware of how the changes in your breathing affect your moods and levels of physical comfort. When you can use the breath as a kind of barometer and window into your bodymind your behavior will begin to align with the wisdom of this aphorism.

Hand:
- Yoga Asana Posture: Bal-asana (Child Pose) supports unsullied reflective qualities of the True Mind.

- Yoga Dhyana Meditation: Asana: **Chair Pose**; Mudra: **Silent**; Chakra: **2nd Swadhisthana**; Visualize: **Upturned crescent shape or the color silver**; Mantram: **Vam**.

Heart: We are products of the earth. We are its breath. When we breathe, the earth breathes. This is the whole heart of the aphorism.

APHORISM NUMBER 51

As the True Mind emerges,
The consensual differentiation between
Inhalation and exhalation
Melts away.

Mind: Even the contrasting breath is seen in its unity when in the presence of the True Mind. At this point in the Seer's development, his relationship to the act of breathing is forever changed. Rather than seeing the breath as a single rhythm of in and out breaths, he comes to regard it as a continuous flow of prana. Then an entirely new type of respiration emerges where the Seer begins to breathe nourishing life-force through every pore of his bodymind. This is known as the True Breath of the True Mind.

Body: Enjoy your work and help those with whom you work to exude a team spirit. This will bring your behavior into alignment with the wisdom contained in this aphorism.

Hand:
- Yoga Asana Posture: Baka-asana (Crane Pose) and the meditation that follows generates a deep connection to nature that is necessary for the emergence of the True Breath.

- Yoga Dhyana Meditation: Asana: **Full Lotus Pose, Stability Lotus Pose, or Easy Pose**; Mudra: **One-finger**; Chakra: **5th Vishuda**; Visualize: **Circle shape or the color white**; Mantram: **Ham**.

Heart: When the True Breath of the True Mind manifests, the Seer becomes a deliverer whose music can remove any obstruction and breech any limitation. He is at once a prophet of life and a justifier of its manifestation. Within this realization is the secret of the aphorism.

APHORISM NUMBER 52

**As it melts away
In the True Mind's light of realization,
Authentic wisdom emerges.**

Mind: When the True Breath emerges it gives rise to the light of realization. In fact, it supports the spiritual function of the True Mind. Bathed in this light, the Seer no longer regards the mind and the body as separate and individual things. In their place, he glimpses the Absolute Mind at work within every corner of the Universe. The cascades of intuition that accompany this stage of mystic progress are staggering by any account. They surpass anything he has experienced before. The Seer has merely to rest his attention on an idea or an object to divine its secrets. Never has the Seer and his soul been more *en rapport*.

Body: With regards your day-to-day behavior, now is the time for overview. If you are involved in a difficult personal situation, step back and look at the big picture. If you can trust in the totality of the situation and regard even the negative aspects as worthy parts of it, then you will vibrate harmoniously with the wisdom of this aphorism.

Hand:
- Yoga Asana Posture: Parsva-uttana-asana (Sideways Bend Pose) and the meditation that follows, supports the wisdom of this aphorism.

- Yoga Dhyana Meditation: Asana: **Full Lotus Pose, Stability Lotus Pose, or Easy Pose**; Mudra: **One-finger**; Chakra: **4th Anahata**; Visualize**: 6-pointed star shape or the color light blue**; Mantram: **Yam**.

Heart: Grasping the heart of this aphorism depends entirely upon your ability to rest within the beats of God's heart. Can you connect to your higher source and rest within its light and wisdom? The emergence of authentic wisdom is, after all, the earth dreaming.

APHORISM NUMBER 53

**When authentic wisdom emerges,
It signals that the player
Is ready to apply the power of
Adroit single-mindedness.
This is musical concentration.**

Mind: Patanjali discusses the mechanics and uses of musical concentration in the third Sutra. For now, he tells us that living the life of a mystic musician prepares us for the real work. Now the Seer has the power and skill to deeply penetrate the True Mind. This is an auspicious moment. The intuition of the mystic musician now functions at a level more elevated and rarefied than ever before. He must do something with it if his progress is to continue. His first choice involves the sensory world.

Body: The act of concentration in the mystic tradition is called *dharana*. It is an important skill to have when treading the mystic path. However, any activity that fosters concentration will support the wisdom of the aphorism. Memorize a list of important facts, learn a new skill, or enroll in a foreign language class. Any activity in the consensual world that requires memory and concentration will support the advanced single-mindedness of the mystic.

Hand:
- Yoga Asana Posture: Sukh-asana (Happy Pose) generates a simple, joyful trust in the wisdom of the universe that supports authentic wisdom.

- Yoga Dhyana Meditation: Asana: **Easy Pose**; Mudra: **Vitality**; Chakra: **1st Muladhara**; Visualize: **Square shape or the colors yellow and gold**; Mantram: **Lam**.

Heart: The divine presence is literally everywhere. If you can take seriously the notion that authentic wisdom is available to everyone, then you will begin to grasp the whole heart of this aphorism.

APHORISM NUMBER 54

**When the player applies this single-mindedness
To sensual experience,
He discovers the ability to disengage his senses
From the exterior world.
His senses, previously tuned to engage the exterior world,
Become aligned to vibrate harmoniously
With his interior world.**

Mind: This is the state where the mystic musician's inner world is in complete harmony with his outer experience. In musical parlance, the Seer is now tuned to play the music of the spheres. At this point the mystic comes to the full realization that he is not a creature of the consensual world having spiritual experiences. Rather, he is a completely divine spiritual being who interacts with the consensual in order to more fully explore his spirituality.

Body: If you want to shape your behavior to resonate with this aphorism, then cultivate an interest in poetry. Make a feast of it and be nourished. It's that simple.

Hand:
- Yoga Asana Posture: Virabhadra-asana III (Warrior Pose III) manifests a spontaneous love of the world around you and those beings in it. A natural extension of compassion towards others borne out of love, rather

than duty, is also produced. The meditation that follows fosters the same spontaneous love.

- Yoga Dhyana Meditation: Asana: **Half-Lotus Pose or Stability Lotus Pose**; Mudra: **Prayer**; Chakra: **4th Anahata**; Visualize: **6-pointed star shape or the color light blue**; Mantram: **Yam**.

Heart: Music, like poetry, is a metaphor that appears, at first, to only describe the workings of the outer realm. But the music of a Seer shows us the true power of a metaphor to reveal the workings of the inner world. Spirituality is the realm of true music. This is heart of the Seer's existence.

APHORISM NUMBER 55

**At this point,
The senses are tuned for the Pure and Silent Song
And readied
For the discovery and complete experience
Of the True Mind.**

Mind: Patanjali now tells us that we are ready for the next step of the mystic path.

Body: Participating in devotional activities will bring you into alignment with this aphorism. Also, it is important that you are able to savor the delight of any moment in spacetime as if it was a devotional activity. After all, from a mystic's viewpoint…it is!

Hand:
- Yoga Asana Posture: Bodhi-asana (Sacred Tree Pose) supports this stage of the mystic's development and prepares him for the complete discovery of the True Mind.

- Yoga Dhyana Meditation: Asana: **Butterfly Pose**; Mudra: **Lotus**; Chakra: **6th Ajna**; Visualize: **Oval shape or the color blue-gray**; Mantram: **Aum**.

Heart: If you can enjoy the journey more than arriving at the destination then you will begin to understand the whole heart of this aphorism.

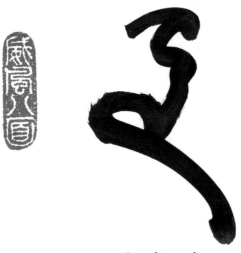

Rajas / Passion

SUTRA BOOK 3

Section on the Gifts and Powers of Music
Vibhuti Pada

This third Sutra deals with the *vibhuti* or "accomplishments" of Music Yoga. These specific accomplishments are also called *siddhi* or "supernatural powers." Within the tradition of Music Masters, they are referred to as the Gifts and Powers of Music.

THE SIDDHI: AN INTRODUCTION

Within the Indian tradition of esoteric music, siddhis are thought of as gifts and signposts along the path that nourish the Seer on his mystic journey. They also provide the Seer with an altogether otherworldly inspiration for his musical expression. While exhibiting something called Complete Musicianship, which will be explained in due course, the musician rests his concentration on an object, concept, or abstract idea. He then expresses that idea musically. An intensity builds between the musician and the idea in the form of a mystic call and response called *Alaap*. If everything goes well and the musician is able to manage the proceeding as it continues to escalate, he experiences the manifestation of an extraordinary ability or siddhi. The ability to fly, instantly understand any human language, produce supernormal strength, or render oneself invisible are among the many gifts Patanjali discusses in his Sutras. The emergence of a siddhi signals a profound accomplishment on the part of the Seer and is an utterly momentous event.

The esoteric music tradition employs a specific regimen of meditations and asana to help bring these extraordinary powers forward. This training method involves balancing the experience of one meditation technique or asana against another meditation or asana. By alternating between the two, the Seer creates a rarefied environment in which the siddhi can more easily manifest. Once the power has manifested, these same techniques provide a way to control the siddhi. For the musician this means spending time before actually playing music to alternate between the two specified meditations or two asana—preferably, both meditation and asana—as a separate cultivation session. This exposes the siddhi environment, which is experienced as flashes of archetypal images, emotions and bodymind sensation. Then, hanging on to the images, emotions, and sensations, the Seer picks up his instrument and applies Complete Musicianship to the specified object of concentration Patanjali describes. If all goes well, the siddhi musically blooms within the mystic environment. It informs the musician's playing experience and takes him to unimagined heights.

APHORISM NUMBER 1

Condensed sound is rarefied and profound.
It fixes your consciousness
By gathering it
To one specific area of your bodymind or
To one specific thing in the phenomenal world
So that its miracles may be revealed.

Mind: To the mystic musician, any event in spacetime is
an opportunity to access and experience metaphysical
knowledge. In order to access that wisdom, the Seer must
disengage normal consciousness and engineer the
emergence of a totally new consciousness that is
designed to understand and make use of the experience.
This is a thoroughly different way of thinking and
behaving that both comprehends and interacts with the
transcendental. But knowledge and wisdom alone, no
matter how profound and life-changing, simply will not
lead to *Mukti* or liberation. Something more is required.
Condensed sound is the musical concentration that
arrives on the heels of this profound wisdom. It is, in fact
an inevitable consequence of mystically driven music.
Patanjali discusses it further in the next two aphorisms.

Body: To access metaphysical wisdom during your day-
to-day activities you must learn to trust in life's wisdom
and power for growth. Avail yourself of any opportunity
for personal growth. Seize the day and watch events as
they unfold. Within that unfolding you will glimpse the
seat of metaphysical wisdom.

Hand:
- Yoga Asana Posture: Virabhadra-asana IV (Warrior Pose IV) is balanced against Adho mukha sav-asana (Downward-facing Corpse Pose).

- Yoga Dhyana Meditation 1: Asana: **Resting Pose, Butterfly Pose, or Easy Pose**; Mudra: **Prayer**; Chakra: **6th Ajna**; Visualize: **Oval shape or the color blue-gray**; Mantram: **Aum**. This is balanced against Yoga Dhyana Meditation 2: Asana: **Chair Pose**; Mudra: **Silent**; Chakra: **1st Muladhara**; Visualize: **A square shape or the colors yellow and gold**; Mantram: **Lam**.

Heart: The heart of this aphorism is concealed within the acts of trust and personal openness. Learning how to surrender to the processes of living and dying and being and becoming will reveal it to you.

APHORISM NUMBER 2

Sound and music,
When experienced mystically,
Harmonize the life of the musician
As well as those who hear it.
It organizes the subtle energies
Of the bodymind
Until the bodymind resonates
With the heart and meaning of the sound.
Then, we may flow into the music.

Mind: The life of the mystic musician centers around the refinement of the intellect that leads to, among other things, preternatural intuition. This intuition does not arrive fully organized from the start. Rather, it exists in a raw and unrefined state. The Seer must employ his musical art to purify this unrefined intuition, which is a vital component of the Atman or "soul." To experience something mystically in this context is to completely deliver oneself to it and rely upon the voice of the soul for guidance. It is a sacrifice of human energy in the truest sense. If the sacrifice is complete and no expectations are foisted upon the mystical experience, the Seer is nourished by it. If not, it becomes contrived and cannot be considered authentic. If, however, it is an authentic experience, it completely changes or "harmonizes" the Seer. Personality, temperament, physicality, and life force all become more organized towards wellness and wholeness. These gifts overflow to people around the Seer and, in a kind of spiritual osmosis, they become more aligned towards wholeness. With the passage of time this harmony intensifies and suffuses the Seer's entire being. Eventually, he merges with the object of musical concentration.

Body: Seeking out physical and emotional security, while endeavoring to enjoy life as it presents itself, will bring your behavior into alignment with the wisdom of this aphorism.

Hand:
• Yoga Asana Posture: Janu-sirsa-asana (Head-to-knee Pose) is balanced against Yoga mudra-asana (Psychic Union Pose).

- Yoga Dhyana Meditation 1: Asana: **Sitting Pose**; Mudra: **Balance**; Chakra: **3rd Manipura**; Visualize: **A triangle shape or the color red**; Mantram: **Ram**. This is balanced against Yoga Dhyana Meditation 2: Asana: **Stability Lotus Pose or Easy Pose**; Mudra: **Centering**; Chakra: **3rd Manipura**; Visualize: **A triangle shape or the color red**; Mantram: **Ram**.

Heart: The secret to understanding this aphorism is recognizing that authentic expressions contain a well-defined seed of decay within them. In order to embrace harmony, one must be willing to accept the inevitable decline of the authentic experience as well as its ascendancy.

APHORISM NUMBER 3

Thus harmonized,
The Perfect Sound emerges from
The Pure and Silent Song
And we are bathed in its True nature.
Then, our own True nature
Can be revealed in formlessness.
We become authentic, integrated, and complete.

Mind: The Seer, having merged with the object of musical concentration, experiences a continuous stream of awareness that circulates between him and the object. Eventually, a single definitive tone emerges from amidst the circulation. The pitch and timbre of the tone will vary from musician to musician, but all experience it as simultaneously emerging from both themselves and an indeterminate place. At the same instant, the Seer is bathed in psychic clarity. But psychic clarity is only a step in the process.

Patanjali believed that liberation could only be attained through a directed approach of experimentation with various states of profane consciousness. Only by experimentally struggling with the un-illuminated consciousness can one hope to understand it well enough to do away with it altogether. In the next aphorism he introduces the method by which this experimentation is carried out.

Body: During the course of your day, avoid jumping into the fray and fixing things even if that's the way you normally handle life. Learning how to leave something "as it is" is a salient feature of psychic clarity. Understanding this will put you into alignment with the wisdom of this aphorism.

Hand:
- Yoga Asana Posture: Sasanka-asana I (Hare Pose I) is balanced against Sukh-asana (Happy Pose).

- Yoga Dhyana Meditation 1: Asana: **Kneeling Pose**; Mudra: **Fire**; Chakra: **1st Muladhara**; Visualize: **A square shape or the colors yellow and gold**; Mantram: **Lam**. This is balanced against Yoga Dhyana Meditation 2: Asana: **Easy Pose**; Mudra: **Vitality**; Chakra: **1st Muladhara**; Visualize: **A square shape or the colors yellow and gold**; Mantram: **Lam**.

Heart: Grasping the whole heart of this aphorism depends entirely upon your ability to understanding the

196

addictive or obsessive tendencies of your own personality. Obsessiveness of any kind is the single largest obstacle to psychic clarity.

APHORISM NUMBER 4

To condense the sound of a singular event;
To mystically express the song of a singular event;
To harmonize the moment of a singular event.
These are the three component parts of
Complete Musicianship.

Mind: A thorough understanding of un-illuminate consciousness is accomplished through the application of Complete Musicianship. In this aphorism Patanjali enumerates the steps of Complete Musicianship:

1) [Condense the Sound] The musician picks an object of contemplation from the consensual world. This can be wind, rain, an idea, or any concept that can be experienced with normal waking consciousness. The Seer intuitively attempts to musically divine the essence of the object. (Explained in the previous Sutra.) Employing his craft, he disengages ordinary consciousness, which educes musical concentration and, guided by intuition, continues to "play the object of contemplation." Soon, the musician becomes harmonized, merges with the object, and manifests the Perfect Sound.

2) [Mystically express the song of the event] Awash in psychic clarity, the player allows his experience to

shape and inform his musical composition. In reality, the Seer proceeds as if he is actually responsible for the creation of the object or event. This creation is achieved with musical notes and rhythm as the musician brings the elements of the event together to give it life; in essence, he is a Pied Piper. He draws on technical music skills as well as emotion, memory, life energy, breath, and intent. Indeed, he behaves as if the object or event would not come into full existence if he fails in his musical endeavors. The player attempts to follow the experience wherever it leads. Whatever he experiences in the inner world is expressed to the outer world as spontaneous musical composition.

3) [Harmonize the moment] The sacrifice of musician to the musical moment builds to a momentum sustained by the diligence and persistence of the Seer. Truly, he presents himself as sacrificial offering to the musical moment. At the same time, it feels to the player as if the moment is approaching him in supplication. If he stays the course and remains open to the musical interchange of object and self, the Seer experiences a fundamental transformation wherein he traverses the breadth and depth of the human condition. Indeed, he moves beyond it and, as a consequence, is changed forever.

It is incumbent upon the mystic musician to "adhere to the terms of the contract" and not abuse the physical setting of his improvisation nor the audience in attendance. If he instead forces his musical agenda, he will never achieve integration. To fully harmonize the moment, the Seer must blend effortlessly with the time of day, the weather and topography, the collective mood of the audience, as well as the gifts and deficits he himself brings to the moment.

Body: Acquiring a high level of skill in Complete Musicianship virtually requires that you confront the darker aspects of your own nature. Take some time to have a hard look at your own personality deficits and devise a gentle plan for resolving them. The unloved parts of yourself must be confronted if you wish to successfully employ Complete Musicianship.

Hand:
- Yoga Asana Posture: Virabhadra-asana II (Warrior Pose II) is balanced against Adho mukha sav-asana (Downward-facing Corpse Pose).

- Yoga Dhyana Meditation 1: Asana: **Stability Lotus Pose or Easy Pose**; Mudra: **Centering**; Chakra: **3rd Manipura**; Visualize: **Triangle shape or the color red**; Mantram: **Ram**. This is balanced against Yoga Dhyana Meditation 2: Asana: **Chair Pose**; Mudra: **Silent**; Chakra: **1st Muladhara**; Visualize: **Square shape or the colors yellow and gold**; Mantram: **Lam**.

Heart: The whole heart of this aphorism rests upon your adventurous nature. Employing complete musicianship as a means of fully exploring the consensual realm will eventually yield to knowledge of un-illuminated consciousness, including your own. This is an absolutely vital part of the mystic quest. But it requires a healthy spirit of discovery and the bravery to confront whatever you encounter.

APHORISM NUMBER 5

**If one works hard and
Approaches his music with joy
Then the musical joining will be authentic.
Wisdom, knowledge, and strength
Of all kinds
Will flow.
These are called The Musical Gifts.
They are the wisdom of Raga.**

Mind: The three steps of Complete Musicianship begin and end with intuitive guidance radiating from the soul of the musician. The entire process must be soul-driven and soul-informed if liberation is to occur. But the achievement of *Mukti* is a journey. Along the way, the soul grants the mystic musician all of the skills and tools necessary for a completely transcendental experience of the consensual world. This experience of life is absolutely fundamental to the yogic quest. Simply put, the Seer who does not know material life cannot know spiritual life. Indeed, such a person cannot be a Seer, at all.

Body: In order to bring yourself into harmony with this aphorism, be aware of habitual thought patterns that you

200

use during your daily activities. There isn't any need to change them at this time. Merely become increasingly aware of the robotic parts of your normal behavior.

Hand:

- Yoga Asana Posture: Salabha-asana (Locust Pose) is balanced against Sav-asana (Corpse Pose) in order to help create the best environment for understanding this aphorism. This environment is also excellent for contemplatively listening to Raga.

- Yoga Dhyana Meditation 1: Asana: **Butterfly Pose**; Mudra: **One-finger**; Chakra: **6th Ajna**; Visualize: **Oval shape or the color blue-gray**; Mantram: **Aum**. This is balanced against Yoga Dhyana Meditation 2: Asana: **Chair Pose**; Mudra: **Silent**; Chakra: **1st Muladhara**; Visualize: **Square shape or the colors yellow and gold**; Mantram: **Lam**.

Heart: Subduing your own aggressiveness will introduce you to the whole heart of this aphorism.

APHORISM NUMBER 6

To be a complete Seer
Is to evolve gradually.
Complete Musicianship must be carefully drawn out
Like the notes of scale.

Mind: The meaning is plain. The mystic process of musical training cannot be rushed. One must proceed slowly and deliberately to successfully cultivate the skills of Complete Musicianship. Each is an eternal truth plucked from the womb of the Universe.

Body: Enjoying what you do for a living is the surest way to align your behavior with the wisdom of this aphorism. Surprisingly, this eludes many people. Strive to make your professional and family life as much of a meaningful experience as you can. Don't merely go through the motions. Then, as Patanjali points out, your life will become like music.

Hand:
- Yoga Asana Posture: Ardha nav-asana (Half-boat Pose or Lazy Back Stretch) is balanced against Sasanka-asana I (Hare Pose I).

- Yoga Dhyana Meditation 1: Asana: **Easy Pose**; Mudra: **Balance**; Chakra: **3rd Manipura**; Visualize: **Triangle shape or the color red**; Mantram: **Ram**. This is balanced against Yoga Dhyana Meditation 2: Asana: **Kneeling Pose**; Mudra: **Fire**; Chakra: **1st Muladhara**; Visualize: **Square shape or the colors yellow and gold**; Mantram: **Lam**.

Heart: The key to understanding the heart of this aphorism is hardly esoteric. In your practice of music, yoga—or any endeavor, for that matter—be happy about your progress and your good fortune at doing something you love. Trust in the outcome and enjoy your journey of discovery. Have a good time. It's as simple as that.

APHORISM NUMBER 7

Condensing the sound of a thing or an event,
Mystically expressing whatever is found therein, and
Harmonizing the expression with the (unique) moment
Are profoundly spiritual and soul-driven skills.
They point to authenticity
Even more than inner and outer discipline;
Even more than steadiness of posture and breath;
Even more than disengaging the consensual realm.

Mind: This is yet another injunction for the Seer to allow the soul to come forward and take the lead of his musical life. The notion that the soul speaks through the intuition is also vital to the process. What's more, Patanjali tells us that Complete Musicianship generates more artistic and spiritual authenticity than any of the other yogic methods previously discussed. In the next aphorism, however, he raises the stakes.

Body: To align your behavior with the wisdom contained in this aphorism, extend love and support to someone who is going through difficult times. Help them to become more confident and aware of their own possibilities.

Hand:
- Yoga Asana Posture: Bal-asana (Child or Infant Pose) is balanced against Virabhadra-asana III (Warrior Pose III).

- Yoga Dhyana Meditation 1: Asana: **Chair Pose**; Mudra: **Silent**; Chakra: **2nd Swadhisthana**;

Visualize: **Upturned crescent shape or the color silver:** Mantram: **Vam**. This is balanced against Yoga Dhyana Meditation 2: Asana: **Half-Lotus Pose or Stability Lotus Pose**; Mudra: **Prayer**; Chakra: **4th Anahata**; Visualize: **6-pointed star shape or the color light blue**; Mantram: **Yam**.

Heart: The whole heart of this aphorism resides in spiritual virtue. How dedicated to the mystic path are you? Spiritual authenticity requires the willingness to let things unfold at their own pace. Yet, too often we become impatient and fall back on old habits of gratification. The Seer must resist this tendency. Your relationship with your immortal soul is at stake.

APHORISM NUMBER 8

**Yet, even they are not as authentic
As musically expressing and harmonizing the soul.
That is the Seer's greatest accomplishment.**

Mind: In this aphorism, Patanjali reveals to us the single most significant and undisputed method for self-realization, so far. Namely, this is turning completely inward and applying Complete Musicianship to the workings of our very own soul.

Body: Immediately tackle any problems that arise during your day. Be direct in all of your communications with others and exhibit great purpose and determination. This will bring you into alignment with the wisdom of the aphorism.

Hand:
- Yoga Asana Posture: Paschimott-asana (Western Side Pose, or Forward Bend Pose) is balanced against Sukh-asana (Happy Pose).

- Yoga Dhyana Meditation 1: Asana: **Sitting Pose**; Mudra: **Balance**; Chakra: **2nd Swadhisthana**; Visualize: **Upturned crescent shape or the color silver**; Mantram: **Vam**. This is balanced against Yoga Dhyana Meditation 2: Asana: **Easy Pose**; Mudra: Vitality: Chakra: **1st Muladhara**; Visualize: **Square shape or the colors yellow and gold**; Mantram: **Lam**.

Heart: The secret to grasping the wisdom of this aphorism begins with a question: "How well can you attune yourself to your own soul?" Once you have answered this question, you will truly begin to walk the path of the mystic musician.

APHORISM NUMBER 9

The soul resides in quiescence.
The Seer finds quiescence within his expression
By listening to the silence between the notes
And allowing his music to flow unimpeded.
If he can divide his attention between
Silence and note,
His quiescence will build in resonance
And fortify his consciousness.

Mind: But where do we find the essence of our own soul? Patanjali tells us that we must musically search out the cosmic stillpoint of our own inner being. We do this by listening to the spaces between the notes we create as much as to the notes themselves. And, as we continue to play, we treat whatever we hear with complete mindfulness and equanimity.

No note or space we musically create is any more or less important than any other note or space we create. Each of our eternal truths or our silences must stand alone and be the single most beautiful thing we have ever heard. Then our own musical stillpoint begins to coalesce. It gradually expands to encompass our complete being and strengthens our total awareness. Any state of consciousness that is exposed to the stillpoint of our soul is vitalized in a spiritual quickening. Simply put, it is stabilized and amplified.

Body: In order to resonate harmoniously with the wisdom and message of this aphorism, it is important to eschew negative thoughts as you go about your day. Helplessness, victim-hood, frustration, and meaningless drudgery must all be avoided if you are ever to capture the stillpoint.

Hand:
- Yoga Asana Posture: Danda-asana (Staff or Rod Pose) is balanced against Anja-neya-asana (Crescent Moon Pose).

- Yoga Dhyana Meditation 1: Asana: **Easy Pose**; Mudra: **Balance**; Chakra: **2nd Swadhisthana**; Visualize: **Upturned crescent shape or the color**

silver; Mantram: **Vam**. This is balanced against Yoga Dhyana Meditation 2: Asana: **Butterfly Pose**; Mudra: **Prayer**; Chakra: **5th Vishuda**; Visualize: **Circle shape or the color white**; Mantram: **Ham**.

Heart: The secret is this: reach for positive thoughts when in the presence of negative ones. The momentum of optimistic and positive thinking can change even the most morose life. But you must have the courage to look your own negativity in the face and put it aside.

APHORISM NUMBER 10

**The perfect balance of silence and note
Within musical expression
Carries the Seer's consciousness
Towards ever-increasing levels of quiescence.**

Mind: As the unique qualities of a given state of consciousness are stabilized and intensified, the musician, buoyed up by his own inner stillness, continues to musically express himself. Then, as a consequence of regarding his continuing improvisation with mindfulness and equanimity, the musician experiences a deepening of quiescence that is quite beyond description or rationality.

Body: Throughout your day-to-day experiences, strive to trust your feelings. Approach all situations cautiously and you will begin to resonate harmoniously with the wisdom of this aphorism.

Hand:

- Yoga Asana Posture: Matsya-asana I (Fish Pose I) is balanced against Bhujang-asana (Cobra Pose).

- Yoga Dhyana Meditation 1: Asana: **Full Lotus Pose, Stability Lotus Pose, or Easy Pose**; Mudra: **One-finger**; Chakra: **5th Vishuda**; Visualize: **Circle shape or the color white**; Mantram: **Ham**. This is balanced against Yoga Dhyana Meditation 2: Asana: **Easy Pose**; Mudra: **Vitality**; Chakra: **2nd Swadhisthana**; Visualize: **Upturned crescent shape or the color silver**; Mantram: **Vam**.

Heart: The secret to a full understanding of this aphorism resides in your ability to consistently engineer medial experiences when playing mystic music. Think of it as a purposeful delay in spiritual gratification. Mystic experiences can range from profoundly uplifting to painfully disappointing. Can you manage to tread the middle path even in the face of transcendence? This is the whole heart.

APHORISM NUMBER 11

The secret is this:
Skill in Mystic expression
Begins with quiescence and
Resides in quiescence.
Thus, the soul is nourished
And the consciousness harmonized.

Mind: A mystic approach to music requires silence, solitude, and stillness. The Seer must cultivate skill in all of these areas. Within the Indian music tradition this is partially accomplished through a ritualized and ceremonial nature retreat called a *chilla*. These musical retreats, which usually take place deep in the wilderness, can last anywhere from thirty to forty-five days, depending upon the traditions of the lineage. During that time, the musician plays one scale pattern, one Raga, or one musical phrase for the length of the entire retreat. For ten to eighteen hours a day he only plays that one pattern or phrase, infusing it with as much meaning as he is able. The player encounters many things during a chilla including boredom, insight, pain, anger, joy, and alternating states of mental and physical exhaustion as well as profound exhilaration.

The goal of a chilla is to induce a series of mystical visions. The lessons and individuals met during the course of these visions guide the musician for the rest of his life. During the retreat the Seer attempts to bring increasing levels of metaphysical solitude, stillness, and silence to every note and every moment. When not playing his instrument, he seeks physical solitude, silence, and stillness. He continues until he is able to, in a phrase, acquiesce to quiescence. Then, the soul is nourished and the player's consciousness blends effortlessly with the moment.

Body: During your day, seek to generate feelings of inner solitude and silence. Carry these feelings with you wherever you go. Even in a crowd, attempt to be alone and you will begin to understand Patanjali's words.

Hand:
- Yoga Asana Posture: Tada-asana (Mountain Pose) is balanced against Settu bandha-asana (Bridge Pose).

- Yoga Dhyana Meditation 1: Asana: **Sitting Pose**; Mudra: **Centering**; Chakra: **3rd Manipura**; Visualize: **Triangle shape or the color red**; Mantram: **Ram**. This is balanced against Yoga Dhyana Meditation 2: Asana: **Full Lotus Pose, Stability Lotus Pose, or Easy Pose**; Mudra: **One-finger**; Chakra: **5th Vishuda**; Visualize: **Circle shape or the color white**; Mantram: **Ham**.

Heart: Quiescence is among the loftiest of all perceptions. It generates radical wholeness and abundant wellness. It accesses tremendous power and wise strength. But the secret is this: it cannot be forced. It can only be allowed. This is the whole heart of the aphorism.

APHORISM NUMBER 12

As a consequence,
The harmonized consciousness changes and evolves.
It is transformed
As a continuity of rhythm, sound, and silence
Grows within a field of quiescence.

Mind: What follows the effortless blending of consciousness with the moment is a state that can best be described as an increase in native intelligence. This is a true evolution that takes place free from the influence of other emotional or intellectual constructs. Afterwards, the Seer notices a definite increase in his mental function and the faculties of reasoning. This is one of the first Musical Gifts.

Body: If you want to resonate harmoniously with the wisdom of this aphorism, it is vitally important to be open to new experiences. Avoid pandemonium and reckless behavior. If you try to observe the life around you with a non-judgmental eye and carefully choose your part in it, then you will begin to align your behavior with Patanjali's message.

Hand:
• Yoga Asana Posture: Bilik-asana (Cat or Kitten Pose) is balanced against Trikon-asana (Triangle Pose).

• Yoga Dhyana Meditation 1: Asana: **Chair Pose**; Mudra: **Vitality**; Chakra: **2nd Swadhisthana**; Visualize: **Upturned crescent shape or the color silver**; Mantram: **Vam**. This is balanced against Yoga Dhyana Meditation 2: Asana: **Half-Lotus Pose or Stability Lotus Pose**; Mudra: **Prayer**; Chakra: **4th Anahata**; Visualize: **6-pointed star shape or the color light blue**; Mantram: **Yam**.

Heart: You are the bridge connecting heaven and earth. You create and maintain the bridge through the exercise of creative potential. When you understand this concept you will be very close to grasping the whole heart of this aphorism. In the meantime, don't take things too seriously. Now is the time for foolishness.

APHORISM NUMBER 13

Harmonized consciousness
As an inner world experience,
Changes and evolves
In much the same way
That our experience of the outer world
Changes and evolves.

Mind: To put it simply, the Seer notices patterns and shapes in his thought processes that were previously hidden from him. He experiences a kind of holographic vision regarding the workings of his own consciousness. The intricate connections of experience, growth, and maturation become clearly visible. He even begins to see the holographic nature of the phenomenal world. What's more, he sees it musically.

Body: Supporting the wisdom of this aphorism requires that you live a life filled with spontaneity and adventure. Beware of capricious or temperamental behavior as it will tend to emphasize an emotional state that runs contrary to the esoteric goal of this aphorism.

Hand:
- Yoga Asana Posture: Tada-asana (Mountain Pose) is balanced against Sarva-anga-asana (Shoulder Stand).

- Yoga Dhyana Meditation 1: Asana: **Sitting Pose**; Mudra: **Centering**; Chakra: **3rd Manipura**; Visualize: **Triangle shape or the color red**; Mantram: **Ram**. This is balanced against Yoga

Dhyana Meditation 2: Asana: **Kneeling Pose**; Mudra: **Cosmic Union**; Chakra: **1st Muladhara**; Visualize: **Square shape or the colors yellow and gold**; Mantram: **Lam**.

Heart: The whole heart of this aphorism resides with enthusiasm. The word is derived from the Greek "enthous" which means, "possessed by God."

APHORISM NUMBER 14

How can this be?
Beneath the surface of the world
Everything is music and
Music is the world of the Seer.

Mind: The mystic musician comes to regard all of existence as a symphony and experiences it, not intellectually, but rather viscerally. While an ordinary person might look at a tree and see bark and leaves, the Seer who has musically expressed and harmonized his own consciousness will see the tree in an entirely new way. Instead of bark, limbs, and leaves he experiences the tree as a composition of sound, rhythm, pitch, tone, and—most importantly—silence.

Body: Aligning your behavior with the wisdom of this aphorism requires something that is very difficult for most people to accomplish. Namely, to be honest with yourself regarding your intrigues and personal deficits.

Hand:
- Yoga Asana Posture: Yoga mudra-asana (Psychic Union Pose) is balanced against Vrksa-asana (Tree Pose).

- Yoga Dhyana Meditation 1: Asana: **Stability Lotus Pose or Easy Pose**; Mudra: **Centering**; Chakra: **3rd Manipura**; Visualize: **Triangle shape or the color red**; mantram: **Ram**. This is balanced against Yoga Dhyana Meditation 2: Asana: **Butterfly Pose**; Mudra: **Lotus**; Chakra: **7th Sahasrara**; Visualize: **Lotus-flower shape or the colors of the rainbow**; Mantram: **Hum**.

Heart: The tree that you see with your eyes is one of life's lies. Your intention is to see the tree in its totality, but without mystic training, you will fail. Clear your mind and look past the surface if you want to grasp the whole heart of this aphorism.

APHORISM NUMBER 15

Harmonized consciousness,
Changing and evolving
Within a field of quiescence,
Appears to be songs, notes, and scales
Because consciousness is song, note, and scale.

Mind: Once the consensual world is experienced as music, the Seer, now fully cognizant of the reflective nature of his own awareness, begins to experience his own consciousness as music. Said another way, the musician becomes the breadth and depth of music immersed in a world of music. This provides him with the opportunity to mystically explore the world "of song" "with song." It is through his musical explorations of various experiences that he will attain deliverance from suffering and achieve the spiritual freedom so cherished in the Indian mystic tradition.

In the aphorisms that follow, Patanjali presents a series of directed experiments for the adherent to perform. Each is a mystic exploration and an essential component of the path. Not to put too fine an edge on it, an authentic approach to either yoga or mystic music is, quite simply, impossible without them.

All experimentation is, in fact a journey of discovery conducted within strict confines and directed towards a single outcome. In this case, the final outcome is called a siddhi also known as a "miraculous gift," "extraordinary power," or "perfect ability." However, achieving the siddhi is not the reason for conducting the exploration in the first place. Rather, as the process unfolds towards its conclusion, the Seer uncovers a critical fact and principle.

The perfect ability that manifests merely serves as verification that the journey of discovery is on course. This is advanced mystic research wherein an experiment is conducted, observed, analyzed, and tested. The knowledge gained along the way concerns the innermost workings of a consciousness interacting with the phenomenal world. This knowledge is absolutely indispensable to the Seer and his spiritual quest.

Body: You must bring a sense of balance and equilibrium to your daily life if you want to resonate harmoniously with the wisdom of this aphorism. Seek out clarity and order in all activities and circumstances. Likewise, a confident attitude will lead to the self-assurance necessary for leading a life devoted to mystic exploration via music.

Hand:
- Yoga Asana Posture: Sasanka-asana I (Hare Pose I) is balanced against Danda-asana (Staff or Rod Pose) in order to help create the best environment for managing the evolution of a harmonized consciousness. In essence, these two asana as well as the two meditations that follow, provide a general foundation for mystic exploration in both the esoteric music and hatha yoga traditions.

- Yoga Dhyana Meditation 1: Asana: **Kneeling Pose**; Mudra: **Fire**; Chakra: **1st Muladhara**; Visualize: **Square shape or the colors yellow and gold**; Mantram: **Lam**. This is balanced against Yoga Dhyana Meditation 2: Asana: **Easy Pose**; Mudra: **Balance**; Chakra: **2nd Swadhisthana**; Visualize: **Upturned crescent shape or the color silver**; Mantram: **Vam**.

Heart: The spiritual path of the mystic requires a rather uncompromising attitude regarding his discipline. Yet, at the same time, if the work is to produce a total experience of the phenomenal realm, the musician must also be accommodating with all that he encounters along the way. That is to say, explorations of any kind have good moments and bad ones. The mystic must learn to take it all in stride and be exceptionally patient. This is the key to grasping the whole heart of the aphorism.

APHORISM NUMBER 16

**By observing the evolution of song, note, and scale
With wonder and awe at what is unfolding
And exhibiting Complete Musicianship,
The Seer intuitively gains intimate knowledge
Of past and future events.**

Mind: All of Patanjali's mystic explorations follow the same template, namely, the application of Complete Musicianship to a specific phenomenon. In this case, by mystically condensing, musically expressing, and harmonizing the spontaneous development of a Raga, the musician generates clairvoyance. In essence, the Seer musically improvises the idea of a song as it begins to develop and gradually continues. Amidst a backdrop of musical call and response with the inner self, the Seer receives intuitive flashes in the form of visions and sensations. These flashes reveal detailed information about past and future events.

As with all perfect abilities, the Seer endeavors to be mystically rational about his clairvoyant powers. That is, he suspends the act of attributing total objective validity to anything he may, or may not, experience. He merely accepts the ability as it manifests. It is, after all, a gift.

Body: Avoid perfectionism regarding this or any of Patanjali's mystic explorations. If you become preoccupied with the idea of acquiring any siddhi then you will not be in alignment with either the message or spirit of the aphorism. In all of your musical endeavors be lighthearted and cheerful. The journey is the most important thing.

Hand:
- Yoga Asana Posture: Vajra-asana (Thunderbolt Pose) is balanced against ardha nav-asana (Half-Boat Pose).

- Yoga Dhyana Meditation 1: Asana: **Easy Pose**; Mudra: **Balance**; Chakra: **3rd Manipura**; Visualize: **Triangle shape or the color red**; Mantram: **Ram**. This is balanced against Yoga Dhyana Meditation 2: Asana: **Butterfly Pose**; Mudra: **One-finger**; Chakra: **6th Ajna**; Visualize: **Oval shape or the color blue-gray;** Mantram: **Aum**.

Heart: The whole heart of this aphorism relies heavily upon your realistic attitude regarding clairvoyance. If you can casually accept the possibility without becoming overtly serious about it, then you will be on your way to turning mystic intention into reality.

APHORISM NUMBER 17

Words as labels and symbols
Become entwined with
Words as sounds and things.
Bathing this confusion
In the light of Complete Musicianship
Allows the Seer to understand any earthly
language.

Mind: Too often, we confuse written or spoken words with the ideas they are intended to represent. For example, when we read the word "thirsty" our bodymind reacts as if we do, indeed, need a drink of water. We may read hateful words in a newspaper and, though they are merely arrangements of ink upon paper, we often find ourselves exhibiting a measurable physiologic reaction to them; our pulse quickens, we breathe faster, and we experience the emotion of anger. As the now famous saying goes, the menu is not the meal. Yet, too often we react as if it is. By mystically condensing, musically expressing, and harmonizing the interplay of words with reality, the Seer generates the ability to communicate with anyone, even if that person speaks another language. In essence, the mystic musician plays language and, as a result, is able to talk with the world.

Body: Attempt to shape your language to be operationally correct and you will resonate with the wisdom of this aphorism. Rather than saying, for example, "Chocolate ice cream is better than vanilla," say instead, "In my opinion, chocolate ice cream seems better than vanilla."

Hand:

- Yoga Asana Posture: Anahata-asana (Heart Pose) is balanced against Baka-asana (Crane Pose).

- Yoga Dhyana Meditation 1: Asana: **Half-Lotus Pose or Stability Lotus Pose**; Mudra: **Prayer**; Chakra: **4th Anahata**; Visualize: **6-pointed star shape or the color light blue**; Mantram: **Yam**. This is balanced against Yoga Dhyana Meditation 2: Asana: **Full Lotus Pose, Stability Lotus Pose, or Easy Pose**; Mudra: **One-finger**; Chakra: **5th Vishuda**; Visualize: **Circle shape or the color white**; Mantram: **Ham**.

Heart: Think of language, either written or spoken, as something valuable. Words are treasures. Their use is affluence. Treat them as if they are delicate gold coins and you will begin to glimpse the whole heart of this aphorism.

APHORISM NUMBER 18

**Exhibiting Complete Musicianship
And playing the mental impressions
Left on the mind
Grants the Seer knowledge of past incarnations.**

Mind: All past experience and mental activity leaves its mark upon our bodymind. A lifetime of experience produces a complex interwoven matrix of these marks or impressions. Employing this matrix of life impression as the inspiration for musical improvisation, the Seer, guided by the discipline of Complete Musicianship, becomes aware of the details of his own past lives and the past lives of others. Those in attendance will, as a result of being exposed to the Seer's musical creation, also glimpse details of their own past incarnations.

Body: To put it simply, love life. This will bring you into complete alignment with the wisdom of this aphorism.

Hand:
• Yoga Asana Posture: Tada-asana (Mountain Pose) is balanced against Anahata-asana (Heart Pose).

- Yoga Dhyana Meditation 1: Asana: **Sitting Pose**; Mudra: **Centering**; Chakra: **3rd Manipura**; Visualize: **Triangle shape or the color red**; Mantram: **Ram**. This is balanced against Yoga Dhyana Meditation 2: Asana: **Half-Lotus Pose or Stability Lotus Pose**; Mudra: **Prayer**; Chakra: **4th Anahata**; Visualize: **6-pointed star shape or the color light blue**; Mantram: **Yam**.

Heart: Courage, vitality, and passion form the heart of this aphorism. If you can devote yourself to the experience of a past life, you will glimpse Patanjali's esoteric message.

APHORISM NUMBER 19

Exhibiting Complete Musicianship
And playing the habits, perceptions, or characteristics
Of another person,
The Seer intuitively gains intimate knowledge
Of their consciousness.

Mind: By employing the stable and readily observable personality traits of another person as the inspiration for musical creation, the Seer is able to superficially join with their waking conscious mind. In effect, the musician will instantly know how a person will react in almost any situation. The psychic depth and clarity produced by the merging is, of course, dependent upon the level of Complete Musicianship the Seer is able to bring to the moment.

Body: Throughout your day, strive to avoid intolerance and realize your own personal limitations. If you can arrange your daily activities to be even and manageable, then you will begin to align your behavior with this aphorism.

Hand:
• Yoga Asana Posture: Surya Namaskar (Sun Salutation) creates the best environment for this extraordinary power to manifest.

• Yoga Dhyana Meditation 1: Asana: **Standing Pose**; Mudra: **Prayer**; Chakra: **2nd Swadhisthana**; Visualize: **Upturned crescent shape or the color silver**; Mantram: **Vam**. This is balanced against Yoga Dhyana Meditation 2: Asana: **Chair Pose**; Mudra: **Silent**; Chakra: **1st Muladhara**; Visualize: **Square shape or the colors yellow and gold**; Mantram: **Lam**.

Heart: Peering into the consciousness of another often requires great stamina as well as detachment. The Seer that is invested in acquiring this siddhi or gets wrapped up in what he encounters, will never understand the heart of this aphorism.

APHORISM NUMBER 20

However,
The Seer does not gain knowledge
Regarding the roots that nourish and support
The habits, perceptions, and characteristics.

Mind: This is a continuation of the previous aphorism. Playing the habits of another will grant the mystic musician intuitive knowledge of their future behavior. It does not, however, reveal the deep inner workings of the conscious mind nor the matrix of mental impressions that make up its source.

Body: Removing clutter and excess from your life will bring you into harmonious relationship with this aphorism. Old clothes, for example, that you no longer wear can be donated to the needy. Clearing out the basement or garage will also support an understanding of Patanjali's message.

Hand:

- Yoga Asana Posture: Since this aphorism follows from the previous one Surya Namaskar "Sun Salutation" is indicated.

- Yoga Dhyana Meditation: Asana: **Standing Pose**; Mudra: **Prayer**; Chakra: **2nd Swadhisthana**; Visualize: **Upturned crescent shape or the color silver**; Mantram: **Vam**.

Heart: The key to understanding this injunction regarding the previous aphorism rests with an intuitive understanding of our inner and outer lives. Within the esoteric tradition of Indian music Masters, Patanjali's words are regarded as a warning to avoid the perils of spiritual materialism. Appreciating the relationship between your inner and outer worlds is the true source of spiritual knowledge and abundance.

APHORISM NUMBER 21

**By exhibiting Complete Musicianship
And playing the shape and form
Of the entire bodymind,
The Seer gains control over the interaction
Of light with the eye
And becomes invisible.**

Mind: Choosing the totality of the bodymind as it exists in consensual space is a favorite experiment among mystic musicians. The corporeal self is seen as a vessel of the soul. Furthermore, this vessel rests in space in much the same way as a boat rests upon the surface of body of water. Like the shape of the boat, the bodymind displaces the air and interrupts the otherwise smooth surface of space by its presence. Attention is called to it. It reflects light and absorbs sound. By exhibiting the discipline of Complete Musicianship and choosing the bodymind's interruption of smooth space as inspiration, the Seer becomes invisible.

Body: In order to align your behavior with the wisdom of this aphorism, it is important to draw clear lines wherever you go and whatever you do. Based upon your own informed evaluation, set definitive boundaries and adhere to them assiduously.

Hand:
- Yoga Asana Posture: Yoga mudra-asana (Psychic Union Pose) is balanced against Ardha nav-asana (Half-boat Pose or Lazy Back Stretch).

- Yoga Dhyana Meditation 1: Asana: **Stability Lotus Pose or Easy Pose**; Mudra: **Centering**; Chakra: **3rd Manipura**; Visualize: **Triangle shape or the color red**; Mantram: **Ram**. This is balanced against Yoga Dhyana Meditation 2: Asana: **Easy Pose**; Mudra: **Balance**; Chakra: **3rd Manipura**; Visualize: **Triangle shape or the color red**; Mantram: **Ram**.

Heart: The key to grasping the full meaning of this aphorism resides in the concept of stability and structure. This is the source of real human power that will allow the siddhi to manifest.

APHORISM NUMBER 22

**Likewise, the senses
Of touch, smell, hearing, taste, and sensation
May be rendered transparent and manipulated by
Exhibiting Complete Musicianship
On their function and relationship.**

Mind: Achieving sensory control through improvisational music depends upon the ability of the musician to peer deeply within himself and view the intricate workings of each sense. Once the Seer is able to intuitively know the heart of each sense, he is able to employ it as an object of musical exploration. The transparency mentioned in the aphorism is existential in nature. Said another way, knowing precisely how the senses work and how he interacts with each, gives the Seer complete control over them.

225

Body: In order to resonate with this aphorism, it is important to consistently follow your aspirations and goals. Be disciplined when striving to achieve your dreams.

Hand:
- Yoga Asana Posture: Surya Namaskar (Sun Salutation) creates the best environment for this extraordinary power to manifest.

- Yoga Dhyana Meditation 1: Asana: **Standing Pose**; Mudra: **Lotus**; Chakra: **4th Anahata**; Visualize: **6-pointed star shape or the color light blue**; Mantram: **Yam**. This is balanced against Yoga Dhyana Meditation 2: Asana: **Full Lotus Pose, Stability Lotus Pose, or Easy Pose**; Mudra: **One-finger**; Chakra: **5th Vishuda**; Visualize: **Circle shape or the color white**; Mantram: **Ham**.

Heart: The key to grasping the heart of this aphorism is this: think of the sensory organs as things that interrupt the natural flow of the phenomenal world. It's as if the ear dips into the flowing stream of the natural world to hear the sounds in it. Regarding all of the senses in this way will reveal the whole heart of this aphorism.

APHORISM NUMBER 23
Exhibiting Complete Musicianship
While playing the momentum of deeds and actions,
The Seer gains divinatory prowess

And the ability to instantly see
The scope and scale of his life
From its beginning to its end.

Mind: Musically seeing into the unknown is but one of the historic gifts of the Seer. This includes, but is not limited to:

- Psychometry: intuitively receiving information from physical objects.
- Hydromancy: divining the future via flowing water.
- Austromancy: interpreting the outcome of future events by wind movement.
- Apantomancy: forecasting the future from chance meetings with birds and animals.

Even the neighing and stomping of horses, if exposed to music guided by Complete Musicianship, can reveal the outcome of future events.

More importantly, however, is the ability of the mystic to see into the depth of his own existence. It begins with the Seer holding an honest appraisal of his own life at the forefront of his mind. If he can successfully employ these memories and experiences as the inspirational source of his musical creation, then he will see the totality of his past and future influence upon the world. At its peak, this siddhi will grant him knowledge regarding the time and place of his spiritual awakening. Likewise, it will also reveal to him specific knowledge concerning the situation of his own corporeal death.

Body: Conflicts arise during the normal course of life. To align personal behavior with the wisdom of this aphorism is to resolve those conflicts in a fair and balanced way. Serenity should be the key. That is, any solution to a conflict should grant all concerned with a feeling of deep relaxation.

Hand:

- Yoga Asana Posture: Danda-asana (Staff or Rod Pose) should be balanced against Ananta-vajra-asana (Eternal Thunderbolt Pose).

- Yoga Dhyana Meditation 1: Asana: **Easy Pose**; Mudra: **Balance**; Chakra: **2nd Swadhisthana**; Visualize: **Upturned crescent shape or the color silver**; Mantram: **Vam**. This is balanced against Yoga Dhyana Meditation 2: Asana: **Kneeling Pose**; Mudra: **Cosmic Union**; Chakra: **2nd Swadhisthana**; Visualize: **Upturned crescent shape or the color silver**; Mantram: **Vam**.

Heart: The secret of this aphorism lay in your willingness to experience ordinary perception in an entirely non-ordinary way. So much of our interaction with the consensual world resembles a kind of metaphysical combat wherein we cross swords with our experience. This can lead to a kind of psychic ambivalence regarding our place within the Universe. If we can learn to "put our weapons down" and authentically touch the phenomenal realm, the whole heart of this aphorism is within our grasp.

APHORISM NUMBER 24

Exhibiting Complete Musicianship
While playing joy, friendliness, and compassion,
The Seer radiates their power and force.

Mind: This musical experiment hardly requires any explanation. What is noteworthy are the stories of past Music Masters who manifested the Siddhi of Radiance. Through their presence alone they resolved conflicts, healed disease, inspired others to great accomplishment, and even controlled the natural world. Some exuded so much joy that they were reported to have physically given off great throws of bright light.

Body: Bringing your bodymind into alignment with this aphorism is simple: be positive, loving, and optimistic as you go about your day. Greet everyone you meet with a smile and kind word.

Hand:
- Yoga Asana Posture: Baddha kona-asana (Cobbler's Pose) is balanced against Surya Namaskar (Sun Salutation).

- Yoga Dhyana Meditation 1: Asana: **Half-Lotus Pose or Stability Lotus Pose**; Mudra: **Prayer**; Chakra: **4th Anahata**; Visualize: **6-pointed star shape or the color light blue**; Mantram: **Yam**. This is balanced against Yoga Dhyana Meditation 2: Asana: **Standing Pose**; Mudra: **Cosmic Union**; Chakra: **7th Sahasrara**; Visualize: **Lotus-flower**

shape or the colors of the rainbow; Mantram:
Hum.

Heart: Your ability to exude a state of balance and quiet repose forms the key to unlocking the secrets of the aphorism. The whole heart of it resides within thoughtfulness for all the people and creatures of the world.

APHORISM NUMBER 25

Exhibiting Complete Musicianship
While playing the powers of animals and things
In the natural world,
The Seer is able to acquire and radiate those powers.

Mind: The meaning of this aphorism is abundantly clear. Simply put, when the Seer plays the strength of the elephant or the gracefulness of the crane, he manifests increased physical strength and exceptional gracefulness. Choosing the suppleness of bamboo as the source of musical inspiration imbues the musician with more flexibility. Musically exploring the nature of wind endows the musician with the ability to rapidly traverse great distances.

Any quality from the natural world may be used as the object of musical contemplation. Of course, merely using that attribute for inspired playing isn't enough. The secret is inspired musical improvisation guided by the discipline of Complete Musicianship. That is the important part of the equation in all of Patanjali's experiments.

Body: Maintaining objectivity in your dealings with others is the key to building a life that resonates with this siddhi. In effect, maintain a healthy intellectual distance from everyday circumstances as they occur. Treat them as delicate things and allow each to unfold without any interference.

Hand:
- Yoga Asana Posture: Balance Yoga mudra-asana (Psychic Union Pose) against Baddha kona-asana (Cobbler's Pose).

- Yoga Dhyana Meditation 1: Asana: **Stability Lotus Pose or Easy Pose**; Mudra: **Centering**; Chakra: **3rd Manipura**; Visualize: **Triangle shape or the color red**; Mantram: **Ram**. This is balanced against Yoga Dhyana Meditation 2: Asana: **Half-Lotus Pose or Stability Lotus Pose**; Mudra: **Prayer**; Chakra: **4th Anahata**; Visualize: **6-pointed star shape or the color light blue**; Mantram: **Yam**.

Heart: The whole heart of this aphorism is, in a word, practicality. Allow yourself to be guided by the force and wonder of the natural world. Respond accordingly. This is not a theoretical endeavor alone. It is also an act of inspiration in which you let the wonders of the natural world take possession of you. When nature expresses itself through your music, you will grasp the secret of this aphorism.

APHORISM NUMBER 26

Exhibiting Complete Musicianship
With an emphasis on mystically expressing
The Holy Light within the mind
The Seer intuitively gains intimate knowledge
The subtle, the concealed, and the distant.

Mind: The experiment extends the powers of sensory perception from the physical to the super-physical. When our senses normally interact with our environment, it causes a certain kind of mental activity that is often described as "luminous." Think of it as the sustained light of discovery related specifically to the senses. For example, smells activate our hidden memories and sight informs our movements and sense of balance. Our sense of hearing constantly reaches out to absorb and interact with all manner of sounds. The subtle processing of the consciousness that is responsible for categorizing, regulating, and using this sense data is the luminous Holy Light.

When the Seer chooses this luminosity as the source of his musical exploration, he acquires the ability to see, hear, touch, smell, and touch the world in a preternatural way. He is able to "see into" an object down to the cellular level or touch an object that is literally, thousands of miles away. In short, the Seer is granted the ability to make contact with the hidden side of life. This, the siddhi of clairsentience, is how a mystic musician explores his world and educates himself.

Body: It is absolutely essential to avoid confusion,

mental agitation, and stress if you are to bring your behavior into alignment with the siddhi described in this aphorism. Also, you should engage in long periods of silent contemplation. It is in silence that the mystic musician learns his craft.

Hand:
- Yoga Asana Posture: Trikon-asana (Triangle Pose) is balanced against Bal-asana (Child or Infant Pose).

- Yoga Dhyana Meditation 1: Asana: **Half-Lotus Pose or Stability Lotus Pose**; **Prayer**; Chakra: **4th Anahata**; Visualize: **6-pointed star shape or the color light blue**; Mantram: **Yam**. This is balanced against Yoga Dhyana Meditation 2: Asana: **Chair Pose**; Mudra: **Silent**; Chakra: **2nd Swadhisthana**; Visualize: **Upturned crescent shape or the color silver**; Mantram: **Vam**.

Heart: Finding just the right proportions of the asana and meditations detailed in the previous section is the key to grasping the whole heart of this aphorism. Likewise, balancing periods of silent contemplation with musical activity is essential to understanding the wonder of clairsentience.

APHORISM NUMBER 27

Exhibiting Complete Musicianship
While playing the wonders of the Sun,
The Seer is granted intimate knowledge of the

Structure, parts, and workings
Of the solar system.

Mind: This experiment allows the mystic musician intuitive access to astronomical understanding. In this way, mystics have had specific knowledge of planetary rings, double stars and other heavenly phenomenon for thousands of years before the scientific instruments existed to see them. Indeed, throughout human history, it has been the mystic that has recognized the significance of the celestial realm and recorded the dynamics of the physical Universe.

To properly educe this siddhi, the musician must come to a visceral understanding of the all important part the sun plays in the life of our planet. Furthermore, the Seer must reflect on the movement of the earth in relation to the sun. Literally, every living thing on the earth exists at the behest of the sun and its regular perambulation across the sky. It is this fact that must form the basis of the Seer's musical improvisation. What follows is wisdom related to the component parts of our solar system.

Body: It is the fear of living an authentic life that separates man from his environment. Said another way, to understand one's place in the universe takes an understanding of the flow of life. A life truly lived and savored aligns the bodymind with the wisdom of this aphorism and the siddhi it details.

Hand:
• Yoga Asana Posture: Adho mukha svan-asana II (Downward-facing Dog II or Three-Legged Dog) is balanced against Marichy-asana (Sage Twist).

- Yoga Dhyana Meditation 1: Asana: **Kneeling Pose**; Mudra: **Diamond**; Chakra: **7th Sahasrara**; Visualize: **Lotus-flower shape or the colors of the rainbow**; Mantram: **Hum**. This is balanced against Yoga Dhyana Meditation 2: Asana: **Resting Pose, Butterfly Pose, or Easy Pose**; Mudra: **Centering**; Chakra: **6th Ajna**; Visualize: **Oval shape or the color blue-gray**; Mantram: **Aum**.

Heart: Confronting the truth of one's own ephemeral nature is the key to understanding the whole heart of this aphorism.

APHORISM NUMBER 28

Exhibiting Complete Musicianship
While playing the shining moon,
The Seer is granted intimate knowledge
Concerning the patterns of celestial arrangement.

Mind: While the previous musical experiment produced knowledge about the specific component parts of the physical universe, this experiment reveals the wonders of celestial organization and alignment. Here, intuitive wisdom concerning the relationship between the moon, stars, and humanity is revealed. The knowledge that follows concerns the effects that fixed stars in the celestial realm have on the human system.

Body: You may align your behavior with this aphorism by eschewing impatience and allowing time to work for you.

This takes a native understanding of the natural processes of growth and change. Simply put, allow the energy of circumstances to run its course. Also, do something positive to promote your emotional or physical wellness.

Hand:
- Yoga Asana Posture: Parsva-uttana-asana (Sideways Bend Pose) is balanced against Bodhi-asana (Sacred Tree Pose).

- Yoga Dhyana Meditation 1: Asana: **Full Lotus Pose, Stability Lotus Pose, or Easy Pose**; Chakra: **One-finger**; Chakra: **4th Anahata**; Visualize: **6-pointed star shape or the color light blue**; Mantram: **Yam**. This is balanced against Yoga Dhyana Meditation 2: Asana: **Butterfly Pose**; Mudra: **Lotus**; Chakra: **6th Ajna**; Visualize: **Oval shape or the color blue-gray**; Mantram: **Aum**.

Heart: The key to unlocking the secret wisdom of this aphorism and inducing the siddhi it discusses rests in a cautious and moderate approach in all phases of your life. Ultimately, this leads one to treat their life with great care and respect.

APHORISM NUMBER 29

Exhibiting Complete Musicianship
While playing the fixed nature of the pole-star,
The Seer is granted intimate knowledge
Concerning the patterns of celestial movement.

Mind: Aphorism twenty-seven concerns itself with the planets of our immediate solar system. Aphorism twenty-eight concerns itself with the pattern of stars as fixed points of light in the night sky. This aphorism directs the Seer to use the pole-star as the source of improvisation so as to gain knowledge of the intricate movement of constellations. Taken together, the previous three experiments represent a mystic exploration of outer space that has been taking place for millennia.

Body: Building up one's strength and reserve is the best way to align personal behavior with the wisdom of this aphorism. Take the time to marshal your gifts and manage your deficits.

Hand:
- Yoga Asana Posture: Adho mukha sav-asana (Downward-facing Corpse Pose) is balanced against Virabhadra-asana III (Warrior Pose III) in order to help create the best environment for this extraordinary power to manifest.

- Yoga Dhyana Meditation 1: Asana **Chair Pose**; Mudra: **Silent**; Chakra: **1st Muladhara**; Visualize: **Square shape or the colors yellow and gold**; Mantram: **Lam**. This is balanced against Yoga Dhyana Meditation 2: Asana **Half-Lotus Pose or Stability Lotus Pose**; Mudra: **Prayer**; Chakra: **4th Anahata**; Visualize: **6-pointed star shape or the color light blue**; Mantram: **Yam**.

Heart: With regard to a Seer's mystical evolution, the

manifestation of this siddhi represents the calm before the storm. After this stage of development, the Seer will experience an increase in the overall impact of the musical gifts on his personality. Likewise, the momentum of mystic occurrence will build to a near overwhelming speed. Being able to "ride it out" is the secret to fully understanding the whole heart of this aphorism.

APHORISM NUMBER 30

Exhibiting Complete Musicianship
While playing the luminosity of the navel wheel,
The Seer intuitively gains intimate knowledge
Concerning the body's workings and constitution.

Mind: The region around the navel is a trans-dimensional gateway called *Kandastana*. At the center of this gateway is the *Manipura Chakra*, also known as the navel wheel. It is the third energy center of the bodymind. A Chakra, among other functions, serves as an intersection point that joins the astral, physical, and causal dimensions. It also functions as an entry point for astral energy to infuse the physical bodymind and give it life. The Manipura Chakra is especially important because it channels life force energy or prana for the entire bodymind. The prana is then distributed throughout the bodymind by a series of energy pathways known as nadis. Since the navel wheel supplies energy to the entire bodymind, a mystic exploration of this energy center reveals the contours of the Seer's health and wellness. It also reveals the inner workings of the vital body organs including the circulatory and digestive systems.

Body: Joyfully start something new and you will be aligning your behavior with the inner wisdom of this aphorism.

Hand:

- Yoga Asana Posture: Virabhadra-asana III (Warrior Pose III) is balanced against Virabhadra-asana I (Warrior Pose I).

- Yoga Dhyana Meditation 1: Asana: **Half-Lotus Pose or Stability Lotus Pose**; Mudra: **Prayer**; Chakra: **4th Anahata**; Visualize: **6-pointed star shape or the color light blue**; Mantram: **Yam**. This is balanced against Yoga Dhyana Meditation 2: Asana: **Half-Lotus Pose or Stability Lotus Pose**; Mudra: **Centering**; Chakra: **3rd Manipura**; Visualize: **Triangle shape or the color red**; Mantram: **Ram**.

Heart: The secret to gaining intuitive knowledge of the inner workings of the bodymind rests in your ability to recognize your destiny in life. Furthermore, how you use the events of your life to shape that destiny also impacts your ability to "see deep within." This is the whole heart of the aphorism.

APHORISM NUMBER 31

**Exhibiting Complete Musicianship
While focusing upon the pit of the throat
Drives away hunger and thirst.**

Mind: The pit of the throat is the *Vishuda Chakra*. By choosing this area as the inspiration for musical improvisation, the Seer is able to control rampant hunger and thirst. He is also able to plumb the depths of desires and obsessions of all kind. Over time, the mystic merges with the respiration and begins to feel as if he is the very air moving in and out of his own lungs. All of this and more is revealed to the mystic who applies the discipline of Complete Musicianship to this area.

Body: Avoid boredom. Seek to make your day-to-day tasks as interesting as possible and you will approximate the feelings described in the aphorism.

Hand:
- Yoga Asana Posture: Ananta-vajra-asana (Eternal Thunderbolt Pose) is balanced against Surya Namaskar (Sun Salutation).

- Yoga Dhyana Meditation 1: Asana: **Kneeling Pose**; Mudra: **Cosmic Union**; **2nd Swadhisthana**; Visualize: **Upturned crescent shape or the color silver**; Mantram: **Vam**. This is balanced against Yoga Dhyana Meditation 2: Asana: **Standing Pose**; Mudra: **Fire**; Chakra: **5th Vishuda**; Visualize: **Circle shape or the color white**; Mantram: **Ham**.

Heart: The secret to uncovering the whole heart of this aphorism is "upheaval." Contemplate the profoundly liberating nature of the sudden awareness resulting from the mystic experience. Within the altogether life-changing force of the mystic experience resides the key to Patanjali's words.

240

APHORISM NUMBER 32

Exhibiting Complete Musicianship
While focusing on the tortoise-shaped channel (of subtle energy)
Beneath the throat,
The Seer is granted profound safety
And stillness.

Mind: There are many different kinds of life force energy as well as many different energetic pathways in the bodymind. One such pathway is called the *Kurma-nadi* or Tortoise Channel which runs through the center of the bodymind. The life force energy that runs through this nadi is related to the eyes and the sensitivity of the skin.

In the Yoga tradition, the exact location of this pathway within the core of the bodymind is regarded as somewhat transient. Generally, they think of it only in terms of bodymind function. However, within the mystic music tradition, Kurma is also remembered as the second incarnation of Vishnu. Symbolically, it represents the dynamic movement of a living human being. It also signifies the motive force of humanity striving for liberation. The Seer focuses on these ideas, the area just beneath the collarbone, and the channel that runs through the direct center of the bodymind.

Taking these visualizations as the inspiration for his musical creation and applying Complete Musicianship, the Seer experiences a profound stillness. This is his stillpoint and immovable center. Soon this stillpoint expands to encompass the musician's entire being and no external force can move him. He becomes profoundly stable and formidably still. In this state, the Seer exudes resourcefulness, physical safety, and security. The steadiness mentioned in the aphorism extends to mental and emotional activity, as well.

Body: Bringing stability to what you have already achieved in life will bring you into alignment with the wisdom of this aphorism. Above all, avoid directionless activity.

Hand:
- Yoga Asana Posture: Vira-asana (Hero Pose) is balanced against Vajra-asana (Thunderbolt Pose).

- Yoga Dhyana Meditation 1: Asana: **Sitting Pose**; Mudra: **Balance**; Chakra: **2nd Swadhisthana**; Visualize: **Upturned crescent shape or the color silver**; Mantram: **Vam**. This is balanced against Yoga Dhyana Meditation 2: Asana: **Resting Pose, Butterfly Pose, or Easy Pose**; Mudra: **Vitality**; Chakra: **6th Ajna**; Visualize: **Oval shape or the color blue-gray**; Mantram: **Aum**.

Heart: Your ability to translate ideas into specific and concrete actions is absolutely vital to understanding the secret wisdom of this aphorism. The key to the whole heart resides in a steady stream of perseverance.

APHORISM NUMBER 33
Exhibiting Complete Musicianship
With an emphasis on mystically expressing

**The Holy Light under the crown (of the head),
The Seer is granted the ability to see perfected
beings
And witness things through their eyes.**

Mind: Throughout history there have been individuals who have attained spiritual perfection. These are souls who, by their work in the earthly realm, have achieved the highest enlightenment and now reside on the spiritual plane. Occasionally, they take human form to aid mankind, but they still retain their place among the higher planes of existence. These Perfected Beings are called Siddhas.

Cultivating a mystic lifestyle through music, naturally awakens the Chakras of the bodymind. The seventh one known as the Sahasrara Chakra located at the crown of the head. It is responsible for connecting the individual to the ultimate reality. When it begins to awaken, the mystic musician experiences a golden light entering and leaving his bodymind as he musically improvises. He feels as though the top of his head begins to bulge upward. If he continues to exhibit Complete Musicianship, the Seer is projected through this bulge into the astral plane. Upon turning back and viewing himself from the vantage point of the astral dimension, the mystic is able to see an intense nexus of silver and golden light radiating from a place just beneath the seventh Chakra. In the refractions of this light, he sees faces and hears voices and song. Taking this nexus as his object of musical inspiration, the Seer comes face to face with Siddhas and is able to communicate with them. He can ask their advice and see earthly events from their perspective as Perfected Beings.

Body: Dedicate yourself to accomplishing concrete tasks and you will align yourself with the wisdom of this aphorism. Above all, be patient.

Hand:
- Yoga Asana Posture: Surya Namaskar (Sun Salutation) is balanced against Nataraj-asana (Shiva Dance Pose).

- Yoga Dhyana Meditation 1: Asana: **Standing Pose**; Mudra: **Cosmic Union**; Chakra: **7th Sahasrara**; Visualize: **Lotus-flower shape or the colors of the rainbow**; Mantram: **Hum**. This is balanced against Yoga Dhyana Meditation 2: Asana: **Resting Pose, Butterfly Pose, or Easy Pose**; Mudra: **Centering**; Chakra: **7th Sahasrara**; Visualize: **Lotus-flower shape or the colors of the rainbow**; Mantram: **Hum**.

Heart: How willing are you to take the reins and assume responsibility for your spiritual progress? Can you trust in the natural cycle of mystic evolution and not rush things? The answer to these questions will provide you with a clue to understanding the whole heart of this aphorism.

APHORISM NUMBER 34

**If the Seer has led a pure life,
Successfully exhibiting Complete Musicianship
During authentic playing,
His intuitive abilities will become wondrous and**

He may experience the spontaneous manifestation Of all these powers.

Mind: Pure in this case is leading a life informed by, supported by, and dedicated to the practice of mystic music. If the Seer surrenders completely to the mystic musician's way of life, it is possible that all of the siddhis previously mentioned will suddenly manifest en masse. Prior to that, his intuition is elevated to unimaginable heights. Everything that he does is accompanied by direct impressions of divine clarity and wisdom. He becomes enthusiastic about the cascade of visions, sensations, mental images, and concrete ideas. Indeed, the Seer feels God at work within him and comes to realize that, through God, he may know anything.

Body: Throughout your day, suggest to yourself that every doorway you walk through is an entrance into an altogether different universe. For you, this new universe is unknown, yet full of wonder for you to explore and discover. This simple game will bring your behavior into alignment with the wisdom of the aphorism.

Hand:
• Yoga Asana Posture: Parvsa-kona-asana (Side Angle Pose) is balanced against Vrksa-asana (Tree Pose).

• Yoga Dhyana Meditation 1:Asana: **Stability Lotus Pose or Easy Pose**; Mudra: **Centering**; Chakra: **3rd Manipura**; Visualize: **Triangle shape or the color red**; Mantram: **Ram**. This is balanced against Yoga Dhyana Meditation 2: Asana: **Butterfly Pose**;

Mudra: **Lotus**; Chakra: **7th Sahasrara**; Visualize: **Lotus-flower shape or the colors of the rainbow**; Mantram: **Hum**.

Heart: The key to unlocking the whole heart of this aphorism resides in your ability to conquer fear. Fear is an indicator. It shows us the way towards our spiritual evolution. Without it, we would never progress along the mystic path. The intimate experience of God's love at work within us lies just beyond the threshold of our fears. We have only to cross it in song. That is the way of the mystic musician.

APHORISM NUMBER 35

Exhibiting Complete Musicianship
While playing the wonders of the heart,
The Seer is intuitively granted intimate knowledge
Of the intricate workings of consciousness.

Mind: This aphorism further sets the stage for an even deeper understanding of divine intuition. Mystic musicians in the Indian tradition believe that God speaks to us constantly and that we learn to listen to him through our craft. As we are learning to listen, we come to understand that our souls are responsible for carrying God's messages to us. The soul uses our thoughts, mental images, encountered symbols, physical sensations, and dreams to get our attention. More often than not, however, our soul communicates with us via our emotions. And the heart is the seat of our emotions.

When a Seer plays the wonders of the heart, he thinks of it as the conduit to the soul through which God speaks with us. Taking this as his musical inspiration, the Seer comes to intuitively understand the detailed workings of human consciousness. In particular, this intuitional awareness provides reliable knowledge about the essential character of the mind. Furthermore, it reveals precisely how the mind causes alterations in pure consciousness. This knowledge is crucial if one is to still the surface of the pond and experience the True Mind.

Body: During the normal course of our day we are confronted with many instances that require us to make decisions or understand new information. In order to align your behavior with the wisdom of this aphorism it is necessary to deal with these instances in a deliberate and firmly resolute manner.

Hand:
• Yoga Asana Posture: Virabhadra-asana II (Warrior Pose II) is balanced against Parsva-uttana-asana (Sideways Bend Pose).

• Yogan Dhyana Meditation 1: Asana: **Stability Lotus Pose or Easy Pose**; Mudra: **Centering**; Chakra: **3rd Manipura**; Visualize: **Triangle shape or the color red**; Mantram: **Ram**. This is balanced against Yoga Dhyana Meditation 2: Asana: **Stability Lotus Pose or Easy Pose**; Mudra: **One-finger**; Chakra: **4th Anahata**; Visualize: **6-pointed star shape or the color light blue**; Mantram: **Yam**.

Heart: Mystic musicians in the Indian tradition sometimes refer to this extraordinary power as the Siddhi of Self-

Knowledge. Indeed, knowledge of the mind's nature and the inner workings of consciousness is knowledge of the self. The key to unlocking the whole heart of this aphorism is reflected in a firm and rock-ribbed approach to the mystic exploration that Patanjali describes.

APHORISM NUMBER 36

Phenomenal experience is a result of confusion.
The intellect and the Divine Self
Have distinct and separate purposes.
Yet often their separateness becomes unclear.
The intellect exists to serve the Divine Self.
The Divine Self exists of its own accord.
Exhibiting Complete Musicianship
While focusing on their contrasts (distinct differences),
The Seer acquires knowledge of
The Divine Self,
The working nature of pure awareness, and
Spontaneous insight into the truth of all things.

Mind: In normal consensual reality, we tend to think of ourselves as physical beings defined by our intellect, personality, and profession. Even if we ascribe to a spiritual path we invariably think, judge, decide, and process our experience of life as if it is primarily physical. But, in reality, we are Divine Beings who only possess a physical body so that we might experience more of the wonders of God's universe. Normally, because our physical self is focused on the world of

248

illusion, we begin to think of our soul as being wrapped up in it, as well. But this is just another example of self-deception. Our Divine Self does not exist within the world of chaos and confusion. Rather, the soul exists within the peace of God that passes all understanding. And while the soul can intuitively assist us in bringing clarity to our confusion, that's not its job. We exist as physical entities to service the needs of our souls and not the other way around.

The way of the Seer is to assist the soul in its exploration of the wonders of the Absolute. Indeed, our non-physical soul should take the lead of our physical lives. Conducting this musical experiment means choosing the contrast between the soul's journey and our physical part in it as the source of musical inspiration. Under the guidance of Complete Musicianship, the Seer is granted intuitional insight so profound that he may access supreme knowledge of anything he comes in contact with.

Body: Extending unconditional love, fairly reconciling disputes, and being wildly creative will align your behavior with the wisdom described in this aphorism. This behavior will "feed the soul" and encourage it to speak freely and clearly.

Hand:
- Yoga Asana Posture: Janu-sirsa-asana (Head-to-knee Pose) is balanced against Settu bandha-asana (Bridge Pose) in order to help create the best environment for this extraordinary power to manifest.

- Yoga Dhyana Meditation 1: Asana: **Sitting Pose**;
  Mudra: **Balance**; Chakra: **3rd Manipura**;
  Visualize: **Triangle shape or the color red**;
  Mantram: **Ram**. This is balanced against Yoga
  Dhyana Meditation 2: Asana: **Full Lotus Pose,
  Stability Lotus Pose, or Easy Pose**; Mudra:
  One-finger; Chakra: **5th Vishuda**; Visualize:
  Circle shape or the color white; Mantram:
  Ham.

Heart: The key to unlocking the whole heart of the
aphorism is this: take your place in life and delight in it.

APHORISM NUMBER 37

**Amid this cascade of spontaneous intuition
The Seer's senses
Begin to function in an exceptional manner.**

Mind: When the profound insight mentioned in the
previous aphorism first presents itself, the Seer
experiences heightened sensory awareness. Sight,
hearing, the sense of taste, smell, and touch become
hypersensitive. This hypersensitivity can be distracting,
at best, and incredibly painful, at worst. In some cases,
mystic musicians have removed themselves from as
much sensory stimulation as possible. But, the True Seer
utilizes these sensations as objects of musical
inspiration and eventually learns to control his new
senses with music.

Body: Throughout your day, assiduously trust your intuition. Listen to your inner voice and you will naturally encounter your life as unforgettable and nourishing.

Hand:
- Yoga Asana Posture: Balancing Vira-asana (Hero or Champion Pose) against Virabhadra-asana III (Warrior Pose III) helps the Seer manage the hypersensitivity of the senses. This asana combination is a very important tool in the mystic life of a Seer.

- Yoga Dhyana Meditation 1: Asana: **Sitting Pose**; Mudra: **Balance**; Chakra: **2nd Swadhisthana**; Visualize: **Upturned crescent shape or the color silver**; Mantram: **Vam**. This is balanced against Yoga Dhyana Meditation 2: Asana: **Half-Lotus Pose or Stability Lotus Pose**; Mudra: **Prayer**; Chakra: **4th Anahata**; Visualize: **6-pointed star shape or the color light blue**; Mantram: **Yam**.

Heart: Periods of heightened sensory awareness brought on by mystic exploration are nothing short of mysterious. Managing these periods requires a willingness to be led by your soul. This is the key to the heart of the aphorism.

APHORISM NUMBER 38

When this occurs, great care must be taken.
Sensory expansion can be an obstacle
To fully harmonizing the moment.

Mind: Once the Seer gets his new senses under control, his experience of the consensual world changes radically. The simplest food tastes like a gourmet meal. Water becomes ambrosia and the faintest smell can trigger otherwordly visions. In fact, everything can become so transcendent and pleasurable, that the Seer runs the risk of being diverted from his spiritual goals. It is at this time that a disciplined approach to mystical music can redirect the Seer and keep him on the path to liberation.

Body: Engaging in enjoyable intellectual games will help align your behavior with the wisdom of this aphorism. Be curious about simple things and play with your thoughts.

Hand:

• Yoga Asana Posture: As with the previous aphorism, two asana are employed to help the Seer manage sensory hypersensitivity. Bilik-asana (Cat or Kitten Pose) is balanced against Bal-asana (Child or Infant Pose). Alternating between these postures supports both spontaneous intuition and mystic expansion of the senses.

• Yoga Dhyana Meditation: Only one meditation is necessary for supporting the wisdom of this aphorism. Asana: **Chair Pose**; Mudra: **Vitality**; Chakra: **2nd Swadhisthana**; Visualize: **Upturned crescent shape or the color silver**; Mantram: **Vam**.

Heart: Safety is the key to this aphorism. A devout and regular mystical practice will provide the stability and sense of security necessary for fully supporting this stage of mystic accomplishment.

APHORISM NUMBER 39

Exhibiting Complete Musicianship
While letting loose bodymind
Attachments, obsessions, and muscular tension,
The Seer gains knowledge of the breath and
Becomes attuned to the flow of vital energy (life
force energy prana).
Thus attuned,
The Seer may project his consciousness
Into the body of another.

Mind: As with all of the siddhis, this musical exploration is conducted with instrument in hand. By adjusting his posture, physical movement, and mental condition, the Seer first engineers a state of profound relaxation. In all areas, he fosters a sense of balance, poise, and subtle equilibrium. He then takes the sensations that follow from deep relaxation and uses them as the object of musical inspiration.

By applying Complete Musicianship to the sensations of deep relaxation, the Seer is granted intuitional knowledge concerning the full scope of pranayama, also known as the Science of Breath. This allows him to spontaneously mold and shape the act of breathing towards a goal of complete awareness of the life-force, or prana, flowing through the bodymind and natural world. This awareness reveals the patterns, pathways, qualities, and types of prana that constantly move into and out from the bodymind. With continued musical exploration, the Seer learns how to completely manipulate his life energy and the energies of others. Eventually, he acquires the ability to project his consciousness upon a wave of prana and move it into the bodymind of other people. In this way he is able to influence their behavior and perception as well as assist them in solving problems and curing illnesses.

Body: Be optimistic throughout your day and cultivate a sense of confidence that everything will go just as it should. This will align your behavior with the wisdom of the aphorism.

Hand:
- Yoga Asana Posture: Anja-neya-asana (Crescent Moon Pose) is balanced against Settu bandha-asana (Bridge Pose) in order to help create the best environment for this extraordinary power to manifest.

- Yoga Dhyana Meditation 1: Asana: **Butterfly Pose**; Mudra: **Prayer**; Chakra: **5th Vishuda**; Visualize: **Circle shape or the color white**; Mantram: **Ham**. This is balanced against Yoga Dhyana Meditation 2: Asana: **Full Lotus Pose, Stability Lotus Pose, or Easy Pose**; Mudra: **One-finger**; Chakra: **5th Vishuda**; Visualize: **Circle shape or the color white**; Mantram: **Ham**.

Heart: Becoming attuned to the flow of prana requires a simple trust in your ability to do so. In essence, though an important mystical accomplishment, regard this attenuation—in fact, regard all mystic knowledge—with a relaxed and easy-going countenance.

APHORISM NUMBER 40

Exhibiting Complete Musicianship
While playing the movement of energy
Moving through the head and neck,
The Seer gains control over the Udana breath
Allowing him to rise (levitate) above obstacles
And remain untouched by muck, mire, water or thorn.

Mind: Generally speaking, musicians in the mystic tradition recognize ten different kinds of prana, consisting of five major types and five minor. Each is anchored to a specific area within the bodymind and functions from this point. Udana prana, which is sometimes referred to as Udana breath, is anchored in and around the throat and above the larynx. Each prana has an exclusive purpose and responsibility. Udana controls the upward flow of life force energy. It supports and controls the sensory organs. It also nourishes the brain and is responsible for providing the energy of cognition and perception. Udana prana is also responsible for man's relationship to gravity. When the Seer musically exerts control over this prana, he is able to neutralize the gravitational pull on his bodymind and levitate.

Body: Throughout your day, endeavor to enjoy the company and camaraderie of others. This will align your behavior with the energies manifested through the mystical exploration Patanjali describes in the aphorism.

Hand:
- Yoga Asana Posture: Surya Namasakar (Sun Salutation) is balanced against Salabha-asana (Locust Pose).

- Yoga Dhyana Meditation 1: Asana: **Standing Pose**; Mudra: **One-finger**; Chakra: **3rd Manipura**; Visualize: **Triangle shape or the color red**; Mantram: **Ram**. This is balanced against Yoga Dhyana Meditation 2: Asana: **Butterfly Pose**; Mudra: **One-finger**; Chakra: **6th Ajna**; Visualize: **Oval shape or the color blue-gray**; Mantram: **Aum**.

Heart: Traditionally, Music Masters of the past have imparted a warning with this aphorism. Namely, that reveling in culmination will put an end to mystic ascent. Said simply, if you think you've accomplished something great, then your progress will stop. This is true of all mystic accomplishment.

APHORISM NUMBER 41

Exhibiting Complete Musicianship
While playing the energy
Moving through the abdomen,
The Seer gains control of the *Samana* breath,
Allowing him to radiate both heat and light.

Mind: Another prana known as the Samana Breath is anchored in and around the navel. It supports and controls the digestive system and governs the assimilation of nutrients from digested food. Also, it is the activating force of the heart and circulatory system. Consequently, the Samana energy flows through the entire bodymind. Mystic musicians regard Samana as the prana that draws together the various parts of the human organism and binds them together.

The musician takes all of these ideas as the source of his improvisation. He also envisions a small flame burning at the heart of the Samana region. If he is successful, he manifests a heat that is both psychic as well as physical. In addition, his digestion becomes formidable and his bloodstream invigorated. In extreme cases, the mystic gives off a subtle luminescence and actually appears to radiate light.

Body: Whenever possible throughout your day, express your inner feelings to those around you. However, don't become emotionally self-indulgent.

Hand:
• Yoga Asana Posture: Baka-asana (Crane Pose) is balanced against Surya Namaskar (Sun Salutation).

• Yoga Dhyana Meditation 1: Asana: **Full Lotus Pose, Stability Lotus Pose, or Easy Pose**; Mudra: **One-finger**; Chakra: **5th Vishuda**; Visualize: **Circle shape or the color white**; Mantram: **Ham**. This is balanced against Yoga Dhyana Meditation 2: Asana: **Standing Pose**; Mudra: **Fire**; Chakra: **5th Vishuda**; Visualize: **Circle shape or the color white**; Mantram: **Ham**.

This is a very powerful mystic exploration. The energies encountered through the practice of this siddhi virtually require that the Seer employ both the asana and the meditations. This will insure safe progress.

Heart: The secret of this aphorism is revealed in the commitment to be inspired and guided by your own feelings. To bathe in the spirit of your own emotions is to grasp the esoteric meaning of this aphorism.

APHORISM NUMBER 42

Exhibiting Complete Musicianship
While focusing on the air
And playing the movement of sound through it,
The Seer acquires clairaudience.

Mind: The Seer engineers a mystic state in which he attempts to see sound waves moving through the air or Akasa. In essence, he seeks to understand the cooperation between the air and the sound that allows us, as human beings, to hear it. Contemplating this notion while playing the movements of air and sound surrounding the ears results in supernormal hearing. The siddhi that results from this musical experiment also grants the Seer the ability to hear sounds and music in other dimensions.

Body: Avoiding direct confrontation with people and circumstances will bring your behavior into alignment with the wisdom of this aphorism. The process of actively sidestepping difficult situations approximates the energetic feeling that comes from the siddhi of clairaudience. In essence, listen to the sounds of life obliquely.

Hand:
• Yoga Asana Posture: Vrksa-asana (Tree Pose) is balanced against Vajra-asana (Thunderbolt Pose).

• Yoga Dhyana Meditation 1: Asana: **Butterfly Pose**; Mudra: **Lotus**; Chakra: **7th Sahasrara**; Visualize: **Lotus-flower shape or the colors of the rainbow**; Mantram: **Hum**. This is balanced against Yoga Dhyana Meditation 2: Asana: **Resting Pose, Butterfly Pose, or Easy Pose**; Mudra: **Vitality**; Chakra: **6th Ajna**; Visualize: **Oval shape or the color blue-gray**; Mantram: **Aum**.

Heart: Avoid the kind of negative thinking that always leads you to fear the worst. Self-destructive reverie should likewise be avoided. Listen for the next good sound and you will be very close to grasping the secret of this aphorism and the siddhi it describes.

APHORISM NUMBER 43

Exhibiting Complete Musicianship,
The Seer who plays the lightness of cotton down
While focusing on the ether and
The relationship of the bodymind to the ether,
Gains the ability to fly through the air.

Mind: Ether, in this case, are the molecules we call air and its related pranic energy. Contemplating the relationship of the ether to the external bodymind, the ideas of lightness, faintness, and the subtle nature of gossamer things becomes the Seer's object of musical inspiration.

The siddhi that is produced from this musical experiment does not result in flight in the conventionally accepted sense. Rather than moving through the air like a bird, it permits the Seer to bring a sense of lightness and diffusion to his bodymind. Once the gross matter of the bodymind is rendered subtle, the mystic need only think about where he would like to go. In an instant the bodymind of the Seer disappears from one location and coalesces in another. Applying Complete Musicianship to these ideas results in the ability of instantaneous movement through space.

Body: Clearly define your accepted sense of reality as a means of aligning your behavior with the wisdom of this aphorism. Clarify your standards and stick to them. Accept no compromise with your ideals.

Hand:
- Yoga Asana Posture: Sukh-asana (Happy Pose) is balanced against Sav-asana (Corpse Pose).

- Yoga Dhyana Meditation 1: Asana: **Easy Pose**; Mudra: **Vitality**; Chakra: **1st Muladhara**; Visualize: **Square shape or the colors yellow and gold**; Mantram: **Lam**. This is balanced against Yoga Dhyana Meditation 2: Asana: **Chair Pose**;

260

Mudra: **Silent**; Chakra: **1st Muladhara**; Continue to breathe naturally and comfortably while contemplating the lightness of cotton down described in the aphorism. Alternating between these two meditative postures creates the optimal environment for the siddhi to manifest.

Heart: The key to grasping the whole heart of the aphorism rests in your ability to give yourself over to the idea of lightness in fine spun cotton down floating on the winds. See it, feel it, taste it, and touch the idea with your imagination.

APHORISM NUMBER 44

Exhibiting Complete Musicianship
While playing the waves of thought pressure
Moving unseen through the ether,
The Seer dissolves the darkness
That hides the light of the True Mind.

Mind: Individuals in the process of normal cognition produce waves of psychic pressure that exude from their bodymind. These waves extend outward in all directions. They collide with other waves and create patterns of interference. These interference waves feed back onto everyone within their influence. This creates a kind of mental inhibition that actually blocks the ability of people within its range to think and reason clearly. The Seer, as a result of pursuing his esoteric discipline, becomes quite sensitive to this thought pressure and is able to perceive its intensity and direction. Taking the movement of this pressure as the source of his inspiration, the mystic musician is able to neutralize the interference waves and relieve the pressure. This results in clearer thinking for all concerned.

Body: All circumstances move through a cycle of birth, growth, maturation and decline. Yet, too often we do not realize when a situation has run its full course. We hang onto it and wonder why things are no longer progressing. Learn to feel when the energy of a situation has exhausted itself. Then learn how to put it aside and move on. This will bring your behavior into alignment with the wisdom of the aphorism.

Hand:
- Yoga Asana Posture: Matsya-asana I (Fish Pose I) is balanced against Vajra-asana (Thunderbolt Pose).

- Yoga Dhyana Meditation 1: Asana: **Full Lotus Pose, Stability Lotus Pose, or Easy Pose**; Mudra: **One-finger**; Chakra: **5th Vishuda**; Visualize: **Circle shape or the color white**; Mantram: **Ham**. This is balanced against Yoga Dhyana Meditation 2: Asana: **Resting Pose, Butterfly Pose, or Easy Pose**; Mudra: **Vitality**; Chakra: **6th Ajna**; Visualize: **Oval shape or the color blue-gray**; Mantram: **Aum**.

Heart: The secret to grasping this aphorism is hidden in our transient experience of thought. In truth, thoughts never die. We only experience the passing of a thought because of its movement within our minds. Accept that every thought that has ever been "thought" still exists within the akasa waiting for us to retrieve it. Succeed at this and you will experience the whole heart of Patanjali's words.

APHORISM NUMBER 45

**Exhibiting Complete Musicianship
While playing any subtle or gross aspect
Of the natural elements
Grants the Seer complete control over them.**

Mind: This aphorism and the two that follow form a complete esoteric concept. In a previous aphorism (43) the Seer learned to render subtle the gross matter of the bodymind. This resulted in corporeal lightness and diffusion. The diffused bodymind could then be moved to another location at will. Applying this same concept to the myriad non-human elements of the natural world results in all manner of miraculous powers. These powers are revealed in the next aphorism.

Body: Go about your day in an entirely open and confident manner. This will prepare you for the manifestation of this siddhi and the specialized powers that flow from it.

Hand:
• Yoga Asana Posture: Parsva-uttana-asana (Sideways Bend Pose) is balanced against Surya Namaskar (Sun Salutation).

- Yoga Dhyana Meditation 1: Asana: **Full Lotus Pose, Stability Lotus Pose, or Easy Pose**; Mudra: **One-finger**; Chakra: **4th Anahata**; Visualize: **6-pointed star shape or the color light blue**; Mantram: **Yam**. This is balanced against Yoga Dhyana Meditation 2: Asana: **Standing Pose**; Mudra: **Fire**; Chakra: **5th Vishuda**; Visualize: **Circle shape or the color white**; Mantram: **Ham**.

Heart: Self-assurance is the key to unlocking the secret of this aphorism.

APHORISM NUMBER 46

Then the Seer spontaneously manifests
An array of exceptional talents that transcend
The physical laws of the consensual realm.
These are:
1) The power to reduce oneself to atom-size,
2) The power to expand oneself to infinity,
3) The power to become very light,
4) The power to become very heavy,
5) The power to extend the reach anywhere,
6) The power to achieve one's desires,
7) The power to create anything, and
8) The power to shape, control, and fulfill any wish.

Mind: The aphorism is plain enough. These are the Eight Great Powers of the Seer. Each of these powers represents both a physical and a metaphysical ability.

Body: The siddhis that follow represent great spiritual accomplishment. The Mystic Musician is, at this point, fully immersed in the world of rhythm, tone, and energy that is the *Nada Brahma* or "Sound Of God." Literally, the musician's day-to-day behavior becomes the mystic experience.

Hand:
Asana Practice
The extraordinary powers described in this and the next aphorism require a consistent pranic base to be contrasted against if they are to successfully manifest. To that end Surya Namaskar (Sun Salutation) becomes the foundation and starting point for asana practice designed to create an optimal environment for the individual siddhis to present. After a period of creating the sequence known as Surya Namaskar, the Seer moves to the contrasting asana:

1) The power to reduce oneself to atom-size
  Virabhadra-asana III (Warrior Pose III)

2) The power to expand oneself to infinity
  Baka-asana (Crane Pose)

3) The power to become very light
  Ananta-vajra-asana (Eternal Thunderbolt Pose)

4) The power to become very heavy
  Parsva-uttana-asana (Sideways Bend Pose)

5) The power to extend the reach anywhere
  Virabhadra-asana I (Warrior Pose I)

6) The power to achieve one's desires
Sarva-anga-asana (Shoulderstand)

7) The power to create anything
Ananta-vajra-asana (Eternal Thunderbolt Pose)

8) The power to shape, control, and fulfill any wish
Bodhi-asana (Sacred Tree Pose)

Surya Namaskar is balanced against the above asana in order to create the best environment for the specified siddhi to manifest.

Yoga Meditation
Yoga Meditation may also be used in addition to asana practice or as a substitute for it. After a period of performing the following Yoga meditation, the Seer moves to the contrasting Dhyana.

• Yoga Dhyana Meditation: Asana: **Standing Pose**; Mudra: **Cosmic Union**; Chakra: **7th Sahasrara**; Visualize: **Lotus-flower shape or the colors of the rainbow**; Mantram: **Hum**.

1) The power to reduce oneself to atom-size
Yoga Dhyana Meditation: Asana: **Half-Lotus Pose or Stability Lotus Pose**; Mudra: **Prayer**; Chakra: **4th Anahata**; Visualize: **6-pointed star shape or the color light blue**; Mantram: **Yam**.

2) The power to expand oneself to infinity
Yoga Dhyana Meditation: Asana: **Full Lotus Pose, Stability Lotus Pose, or Easy Pose**; Mudra: **One-finger**; Chakra: **5th Vishuda**; Visualize: **Circle shape or the color white**; Mantram: **Ham**.

3) The power to become very light
Yoga Dhyana Meditation: Asana: **Kneeling Pose**; Mudra: **Cosmic Union**; Chakra: **2nd Swadhisthana**; Visualize: **Upturned crescent shape or the color silver**; Mantram: **Vam**.

4) The power to become very heavy
Yoga Dhyana Meditation: Asana: **Full Lotus Pose, Stability Lotus Pose, or Easy Pose**; Mudra: **One-finger**; Chakra: **4th Anahata**; Visualize: **6-pointed star shape or the color light blue**; Mantram: **Yam**.

5) The power to extend the reach anywhere
Yoga Dhyana Meditation: Asana: **Stability Lotus Pose or Easy Pose**; Mudra: **Centering**; Chakra: **3rd Manipura**; Visualize: **Triangle shape or the color red**; Mantram: **Ram**.

6) The power to achieve one's desires
Yoga Dhyana Meditation: Asana: **Kneeling Pose**; Mudra: **Cosmic Union**; Chakra: **1st Muladhara**; Visualize: **Square shape or the colors yellow and gold**; Mantram: **Lam**.

7) The power to create anything
Yoga Dhyana Meditation: Asana **Standing Pose**;
Mudra: **Lotus**; Chakra: **4th Anahata**; Visualize: **6-
pointed star shape or the color light blue**;
Mantram: **Yam**.

**8) The power to shape, control, and fulfill any
wish**
Yoga Dhyana Meditation: Asana **Standing Pose**;
Mudra: **Lotus**; Chakra: **4th Anahata**; Visualize: **6-
pointed star shape or the color light blue**;
Mantram: **Yam**.

Heart: The key to grasping the whole heart of this
aphorism revolves around your ability to surrender to
new perceptions and to act decisively when those
perceptions arise. Immediately employ the mystic wisdom
that extends from them. Said another way, submit to the
siddhi and seize the moment. This is the secret of the
aphorism.

APHORISM NUMBER 47

**As these exceptional talents begin to coalesce
The Seer's bodymind becomes
Graceful, radiantly beautiful, and strong as
diamonds.**

Mind: The act of musically exploring the natural
elements of the consensual world result in the Eight Great
Powers of the Seer. This eliminates karma of all kinds

and gives the Seer complete control over his bodymind. It also allows the light of our natural divinity to shine forth into the world.

Body: During your day-to-day experiences, strive to see things objectively and honestly. This will align you with the wisdom of the aphorism.

Hand:
- Yoga Asana Posture: Surya Namaskar (Sun Salutation) is balanced against Baddha kona-asana (Cobbler's Pose) in order to help create the best environment for this extraordinary power to manifest.

- Yoga Dhyana Meditation 1: Asana: **Standing Pose**; Mudra: **Cosmic Union**; Chakra: **7th Sahasrara**; Visualize: **Lotus-flower shape or the colors of the rainbow**; Mantram: **Hum**. This is balanced against Yoga Dhyana Meditation 2: Asana: **Half-Lotus Pose or Stability Lotus Pose**; Mudra: **Prayer**; Chakra: **4th Anahata**; Visualize: **6-pointed star shape or the color light blue**; Mantram: **Yam**.

Heart: Can you recognize your responsibility in everything that you experience? Understand the cooperative nature of your relationship with consensual experience and you will grasp the whole heart of this aphorism.

APHORISM NUMBER 48

Play the intrinsic nature of the sensory processes,
Including purposes, perceptions, and their partnerships.
Play the act of identifying perception with the self.
Bathe each in Complete Musicianship
And you will be granted total mastery over them.

Mind: This experiment reveals the function of the Divine Self. The senses previously mastered are literally turned in on themselves. The ear, for example, is directed to listen to its own function and the eyes are asked to see themselves at work. Further, the Seer looks to the intersection of the self with the senses and observes himself in the process of sensing the environment. Taking this process as the source of his musical inspiration, the Seer mystically joins with himself in the act of perceiving. This gives him complete control over the sensory perception process.

Body: The best way to align yourself with the wisdom of this aphorism is to connect lovingly with those people most important to you.

Hand:
• Yoga Asana Posture: Adho mukha sav-asana (Downward-facing Corpse Pose) is balanced against Surya Namaskar (Sun Salutation).

• Yoga Dhyana Meditation 1: Asana: **Chair Pose**; Mudra: **Silent**; Chakra: **1st Muladhara**; Visualize: **Square shape or the colors yellow and gold**;

Mantram: **Lam**. This is balanced against Yoga Dhyana Meditation 2: Asana: **Standing Pose**; Mudra: **Prayer**; Chakra: **2nd Swadhisthana**; Visualize: **Upturned crescent shape or the color silver**; Mantram: **Vam**.

Heart: In the search for mystic harmony, the Seer runs the risk of moving too fast and betraying his own deeply held beliefs. Take your time. Conduct all of your mystic explorations without hurry and without worry. This will lead you unerringly to the whole heart of this aphorism.

APHORISM NUMBER 49

From this mastery
You will learn to move faster than the mind
And be able to function beyond the ordinary senses.
You will have the ability to move outside the corporeal body
And will exert control over the natural ground of being (natural world).

Mind: From a now masterful control of the sensory process, the Seer is able to transcend it completely. He acquires the ability to move "in between" the instantaneous acts of seeing and remain invisible to the naked eye. He is able to move between thoughts and hear the space between sounds. The mystic, who is in full manifestation of this siddhi, learns to operate obliquely to normal perception, functionally moving about in a sensory dimension parallel to our own yet, normally hidden from us.

Body: Take the initiative in all of your affairs. This will bring your behavior into alignment with the wisdom of this aphorism.

Hand: The following asana and meditation pairs can be practiced together or separately. Balancing one against the other creates the ideal environment for the extraordinary power to manifest.

Asana Practice

As in aphorism forty-six, one asana forms the first part of a pair of poses that are balanced one against another in order to create the best environment for the emergence of the musical gift. This first asana is Surya Namaskar (Sun Salutation). After a period of time, move on to the second part:

You will learn to move faster than the mind
Sarva-anga-asana (Shoulderstand)

And be able to function beyond the ordinary senses.
Sasanka-asana I (Hare Pose I)

You will have the ability to move outside the corporeal body
Virabhadra-asana IV (Warrior Pose IV)

And will exert control over the natural ground of being.
Ananta-vajra-asana (Eternal Thunderbolt Pose)

Yoga Meditation

- Yoga Dhyana Meditation 1: Asana: **Standing Pose**; Mudra: **Prayer**; Chakra: **2nd Swadhisthana**; Visualize: **Upturned crescent shape or the color silver**; Mantram: **Vam**. Breathe naturally and comfortably for as long as you like. Then, as guided by your intuition, move on to the second meditation.

You will learn to move faster than the mind

- Yoga Dhyana Meditation: Asana: **Kneeling Pose**; Mudra: **Cosmic Union**; Chakra: **1st Muladhara**; Visualize: **Square shape or the colors yellow and gold;** Mantram: **Lam**.

And be able to function beyond the ordinary senses.

- Yoga Dhyana Meditation: Asana: **Kneeling Pose**; Mudra: **Fire**; Chakra: **1st Muladhara**; Visualize: **Square shape or the colors yellow and gold**; Mantram: **Lam**.

You will have the ability to move outside the corporeal body

- Yoga Dhyana Meditation: Asana: **Resting Pose, Butterfly Pose, or Easy Pose**; Mudra: **Prayer**; Chakra: **6th Ajna**; Visualize: **Oval shape or the color blue-gray**; Mantram: **Aum**.

And will exert control over the natural ground of being.

- Yoga Dhyana Meditation: Asana: **Standing Pose**;

Mudra: **Fire**; Chakra: **5th Vishuda**; Visualize:
Circle shape or the color white; Mantram:
Ham.

Breathe naturally and comfortably during all of these
meditations. Contemplate each associated siddhi as
described in the aphorism. Remember, these two meditations
are balanced one against the other in order to create the
optimal environment for each of the siddhis to manifest.

Heart: Following the path of the Mystic Musician is risky
business. It requires the courage to face the inevitability
of a complete change in your life. Accept the risks and
you will unlock the secrets of this aphorism.

APHORISM NUMBER 50

In the presence of the perfect virtue
Of Complete Musicianship
The distinction between the True Mind
And the essential nature of the phenomenal world
Becomes discernibly clear.
The Seer is granted mastery over
All states and forms of existence,
Resulting in fundamental knowledge
Concerning everything in existence.

Mind: Here, Patanjali shows us the promise of the mystic
path. Said another way, this is what we may all become.
The fundamental knowledge mentioned in the aphorism is

universal in nature. It intuitively leads you to the awareness of the Absolute in everything. Yet, at the same time, the Seer acts on this knowledge and brings the force of it into the consensual world. Indeed, the mystic musician, through his craft, channels God's light and love through himself and extends it in an unbroken nourishing stream into the world.

Body: Any activity that fosters sensitivity, devotion or inspiration will align the behavior with the wisdom of this aphorism. Above all, listen to your inner voice and trust in its guidance.

Hand:
• Yoga Asana Posture: Bhujang-asana (Cobra Pose) is balanced against Paripurma nav-asana or Kriya-asana (Longboat Pose).

• Yoga Dhyana Meditation 1: Asana: **Easy Pose**; Mudra: **Vitality**; Chakra: **2nd Swadhisthana**; Visualize: **Upturned crescent shape or the color silver**; Mantram: **Vam**. This is balanced against Yoga Dhyana Meditation 2: Asana: **Easy Poses**; Mudra: **Balance**; Chakra: **3rd Manipura**; Visualize: **Triangle shape or the color red**; Mantram: **Ram**.

Heart: To the Mystic Musician, there is little difference between spiritual tasks and artistic expression. Indeed, he regards them as the same thing. The Seer's life is one in which being true to one's feelings is being true to God.

APHORISM NUMBER 51

If the Seer can remain
Dispassionate and unattached
To this mastery and knowledge, then
The final seeds of suffering and bondage
Will dwindle away.
The Seer will stand alone in trans-conscious
awareness
As the final step towards liberation.

Mind: If the Seer isn't careful, he can become attached to his new role as wellspring of the Absolute. If he can remain aloof, even to his own power, then the final alterations and disturbances on the surface of the pond will cease. The Seer can now see; he is liberated. No more conscious acts, in the conventional sense, will ever happen again.

Esoteric tradition holds that Perfected Beings from the spiritual realms will gather to welcome the emancipated Seer who can now freely walk among them. This is a sign of great spiritual accomplishment.

Body: Muster your talents and skills and do something nice for someone else. Using your gifts for the betterment of others will put your behavior in alignment with the wisdom of this aphorism.

Hand:
• Yoga Asana Posture: Bodhi-asana (Sacred Tree Pose) is balanced against Bilik-asana (Cat or Kitten Pose) in order to help create the best environment for the development

of trans-conscious awareness. As with the meditations that follow, the Seer should alternate between them.

- Yoga Dhyana Meditation 1: Asana: **Butterfly Pose**; Mudra: **Lotus**; Chakra: **6th Ajna**; Visualize: **Oval shape or the color blue-gray**; Mantram: **Aum**. This is balanced against Yoga Dhyana Meditation 2: Asana: **Chair Pose**; Mudra: **Vitality**; Chakra: **2nd Swadhisthana**; Visualize: **Upturned crescent shape or the color silver**; Mantram: **Vam**.

Heart: Arrogance, pride, complacency, dogmatism, and self-importance are not the same as being unattached. This is a critical stage in the mystic's development. Guard against conceit and you will grasp the whole heart and power of this aphorism.

APHORISM NUMBER 52

The liberated Seer must even turn away
From the recognition of celestial beings
Who wish to praise and glorify him.
This temptation
Only leads back to attachment and suffering.

Mind: Even though Perfected Beings gather to pay homage to the efforts of the liberated Seer, he employs his music to turn away from them. For even this last emancipation can be corrupted. If he succumbs to even the slightest bit of ego at his accomplishment, the mystic will once again find himself bound to the world of illusion.

Body: Establishing a lofty goal and working towards it will bring your behavior into alignment with the wisdom of this aphorism. Also, enjoy new beginnings and extend unconditional love to the people and the world around you.

Hand:
- Yoga Asana Posture: Only one asana is needed to protect the Seer and stele him against the ego. Surya Namaskar (Sun Salutation) keeps the ego from disturbing the mystic grace of the Seer.
- Yoga Dhyana Meditation: (At this stage of development, the mystic musician needs only one meditation to keep the ego in check.) Asana: **Standing Pose**; Mudra: **Lotus**; Chakra: **4th Anahata**; Visualize: **6-pointed star shape or the color light blue**; Mantram: **Yam**.

Heart: At this stage of development the mystic musician is rapidly approaching the culmination of his devotional work. This is a delicate phase. Reckless behavior or a wasting of energy through total self-sacrifice will wear down the Seer. Eschew naiveté and you will grasp the whole heart of this aphorism.

APHORISM NUMBER 53

Exhibiting Complete Musicianship
While playing the moving succession
Of the segmented moments known as time,
The Seer is granted discerning transcendental knowledge.

Mind: Instead of accepting the praise of Perfected Beings, the Seer takes the experience of time as the object of his inspiration. Now liberated, he is able to make use of the vast spiritual knowledge that flows to him.

Body: Try to go about your day motivated by feelings of deep gratitude. Be thankful for all of the joy and fulfillment you've ever experienced in your life. Especially be grateful for life's small blessings and gifts. This will align your behavior with the wisdom of this aphorism.

Hand:
- Yoga Asana Posture: Bilik-asana (Cat or Kitten Pose) is balanced against Danda-asana (Staff or Rod Pose) in order to help create the best environment for this extraordinary power to manifest.

- Yoga Dhyana Meditation 1: Asana: **Chair Pose**; Mudra: **Vitality**; Chakra: **2nd Swadhisthana**; Visualize: **Upturned crescent shape or the color silver**; Mantram: **Vam**. This is balanced against Yoga Dhyana Meditation 2: Asana: **Easy Pose**; Mudra: **Balance**; Chakra: **2nd Swadhisthana**; Visualize: **Upturned crescent shape or the color silver**; Mantram: **Vam**.

Heart: The key to grasping the whole heart of this aphorism can be summed up in one word: abundance.

APHORISM NUMBER 54

This knowledge reveals
The subtle similarities and differences
Between things of like nature and appearance.
This is the power of Perfect Discernment.

Mind: Endowed with this knowledge, the Seer acquires near omniscience. Subtle differences become just as clear as obvious ones on the consensual realm. More importantly, the similarities between things are revealed. This is vital to successfully completing the last steps into Eternity. The Seer, having transcended time, now clearly sees the root of all illusion and limitation. The entire world is opened before him.

Body: To bring everyday behavior into alignment with this aphorism requires that you devote time and energy towards an unpopular but righteous cause. However, do not expend all of your energy in complete self-sacrifice.

Hand:
• Yoga Asana Posture: Settu bandha-asana (Bridge Pose) is balanced against Hala-asana (Plough Pose) in order to help create the best environment for the power of Perfect Discernment to manifest.

• Yoga Dhyana Meditation 1: Asana **Full Lotus Pose, Stability Lotus Pose, or Easy Pose**; Mudra: **One-finger**; Chakra: **5th Vishuda**; Visualize: **Circle shape or the color white**; Mantram: **Ham**. This is balanced against Yoga

Dhyana Meditation 2: Asana: **Kneeling Pose**;
Mudra: **Cosmic Union**; Chakra: **1st Muladhara**;
Visualize: **Square shape or the colors yellow
and gold**; Mantram: **Lam**.

Heart: Courage is vital when first manifesting the siddhi
of Perfect Discernment. Be careful and measured when
employing this gift. It is easy to overestimate one's ability.

APHORISM NUMBER 55

**The Seer can look at things and conditions
With a musical eye,
Perceive them
In all of their constituent parts and proclivities,
And is able to separate them
From the reality of the True Mind.
Time, space, and the processes of the world
Are seen in a total and unified ground of being.**

Mind: Liberation is now almost complete. When the
entire world of existence is spread before him, the Seer
is able to clearly see what is the True Mind and what is
not. He initially perceives it as the flow of music when in
the throes of improvisation. Indeed, the very fabric of
creation is experienced as song.

Body: The closest common behavior that approximates
this penultimate stage of liberation occurs when we
express a heartfelt personal need. It seems appropriate,

somehow, that standing up for one's needs is the seed of great spiritual accomplishment.

Hand:

- Yoga Asana Posture: Utkat-asana (Mighty Pose) is balanced against Vajra-asana (Thunderbolt Pose) in order to create the best environment for the "musical eye" to manifest.

- Yoga Dhyana Meditation 1: Asana: **Stability Lotus Pose or Easy Pose**; Mudra: **Centering**; Chakra: **3rd Manipura**; Visualize: **Triangle shape or the color red**; Mantram: **Ram**. This is balanced against Yoga Dhyana Meditation 2: Asana: **Resting Pose, Butterfly Pose, or Easy Pose**; Mudra: **Vitality**; Chakra: **6th Ajna**; Visualize: **Oval shape or the color blue-gray**; Mantram: **Aum**.

Heart: At this point, the Seer's burning passion for music has been transformed into spiritual accomplishment. Indeed, the musician has been transformed, fired within the alchemic furnace of his own will. Only one more step need be taken.

APHORISM NUMBER 56

At this stage
The consciousness becomes as pure as sound itself
And the Seer merges with the Pure and Silent Song.
We are complete.
Nothing else remains.

We are Raga;
We are song.

Mind: This is the final stage of the mystic musician's quest. Here the boundary between the real and the unreal universe is breached as the musician experiences the world in a state of pure reflective awareness. He is informed by the Absolute. He is shaped and nourished by it. God, song, and the Seer himself, become one.

Body: Make music your life. In point of fact, make music *of* your life. Embrace all kinds of musical expression. Listen to it. Compose, sing, and play music in any way that you can. This will bring your behavior into alignment with the wisdom of the aphorism.

Hand: Only one Yoga asana and one meditation are required to vitalize and contemplate this aphorism.

- Yoga Asana Posture: Bodhi-asana (Sacred Tree Pose) is the only asana necessary to grasp the esoteric meaning of this aphorism.

- Yoga Dhyana Meditation: Asana: **Butterfly Pose**; Mudra: **Lotus**; Chakra: **6th Ajna**; Visualize: **Oval shape or the color blue-gray**; Mantram: **Aum**.

Heart: The heart of this aphorism lies in the experience of liberation itself and is quite beyond description in any language.

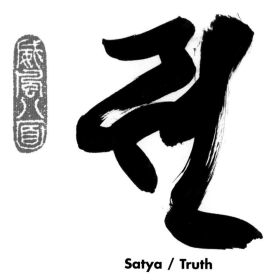

Satya / Truth

SUTRA BOOK 4

KAIVALYA PADA: THE DISPUTED TEXT

The fourth Yoga Sutra is called **Kaivalya Pada** or Section on Complete Release. The first three Sutras form a delineated pedagogical progression that moves the student from the bound world of illusion to the boundless world of the Absolute. The fourth Sutra, however, does not continue this progression. In fact, it backtracks in many ways, providing an almost random assortment of Yoga theory and metaphysical context about the first three Sutras. It also vaguely reframes the information already covered in the previous Sutra. This has led many scholars to assert that it is the work of an anonymous author and was not written by Patanjali at all. This circumstance is not unusual in the world's great wisdom traditions. Additions and modifications have also found their way into many Buddhist, Christian, Taoist, and Islamic texts, to name but a few.

At my current stage of ignorance and understanding, I do not have a firm opinion as to the authorship of Kaivalya Pada. However, within the Mystic Music tradition that forms the basis of this present work, it is assumed that this section was added many years after Patanjali's passing from the consensual realm. Furthermore, it is felt that much of it muddies the water, philosophically speaking. I am content to leave the matter to those interested in scholarly pursuits. Personally, I have a preference for practical information transmitted solely within an oral context. And this oral tradition separates the fourth Sutra from the previous three in several significant ways:

286

- There are no specific asana assigned to vitalize the experience of the individual aphorisms.
- There are no specific meditations employed in contemplating the wisdom contained in the individual aphorisms.
- No clues to deciphering the aphorisms are preserved in this oral tradition.
- The poetic structure and language of Kaivalya Pada is decidedly different from the previous three Sutras.

To be sure, none of this solidly confirms the assertion that Kaivalya Pada was not original to Patanjali. Indeed, though suspicious of its origins, Music Masters still transmit it to their students. In a way, it leaves the fledgling Seer with much to ponder regarding his chosen spiritual path. Think of it as a poetic afterword that reminds the musician that he is always exploring, always experimenting, and always growing.

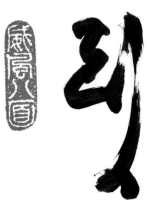

Yana / Spiritual Vehicle

KAIVALYA PADA:
COMPLETE RELEASE

1

Those musical gifts that are acquired
By harmonizing the consciousness
Can manifest spontaneously at birth
If one has cultivated them in a previous life.
They may also be acquired
Through the use of herbs and sacred foods,
Through singing and chanting, as well as
Through mystic experience resulting from ascetic practices.
Sometimes siddhis arise of their own accord.
We do not know the reasons for this.

2

The Seer is sometimes transformed
Into a being altogether different
From those beings around him.
But it is the unlimited field of boundlessness
That transforms all of the natural world.
Authentic music channels the profusion of natural energy
And alters all that it touches.

3

Transformation is a natural occurrence
That does not rely on karma, intent, or previously sown seeds.
Transformation is the way of nature;
Transformation is the way of music.
Authentic music removes obstacles.
It changes the course of rivers and
Seeks its own place of rest.

But it must be cultivated
The way a farmer tends his fields.

4
The tendency to see the self as separate
From the Absolute,
Leads each of us to separate ourselves
From the Absolute.
We may become one entity or many entities,
Depending upon our force of personality.
But we will always be separate from
The Pure and Silent Song.
Authentic music remedies this separateness.

5
How many beings are you?
How many faces do you have?
It doesn't really matter
Because the force of natural energy
Is constantly directing you.
You flow within the strains of the Raga;
You flow from a single source point.

6
Once the consciousness is fixed in mystic expression,
You will no longer contribute to separateness.
Authenticity will reign over the artificial
And you will learn to direct natural forces.
You will learn to ride svara. (tone)

7
Karma is neither black nor white;
Karma is neither good nor evil.
It is a blind force and
The unrealized are affected by it constantly.
The realized Seer is not affected by it at all.
The actions of ordinary people can be good, bad, or indifferent.
The actions of the Seer transcend all three.

8
What is born from the Seer's music
Depends on what is needed most
At the time of composition.
But the Seer remains aloof to the fulfilled need.
He is merely a vessel for its transmission.

9
Memory is active, changing, and alive.
It holds our existence together like a web;
It creates the impression
Of past, present, and future.
Therefore it has the power to transcend
The past, the present, and the future.

10
Past, present, and future have always existed
Because our will to experience the Absolute
Has always existed.
Memory and impression have always existed
Because our desire to know God
Has always existed.

11
Cause and effect are inseparable.
Essence and object are inseparable.
Memory and impression are inseparable.
They become invisible in the presence of Raga
And their seeds are dissolved.

12
Objects in the natural world
Possess an essence and a history.
Each is a gateway into another world
With its own laws and facts of causation.
This world is exposed with music.

13
These worlds,
Though different,
Are part of the natural world.
These worlds,
Whether manifested or unmanifested,
Are affected by natural forces.
These worlds,
Whether visible or invisible,
Are part of the unlimited field of boundlessness.

14
Each of these worlds overlaps with other worlds
And we only see where they come together.
Only a musician can expand this vision.

15
Each person experiences this interplay of worlds differently
And can only see what is meaningful to them.
Only a musician can expand this vision.

16
No one need see this interplay of worlds for it to occur.
No one need be there to cross the threshold of these worlds.
These worlds exist outside the need of experience.

17
An object must cause a vibration and sound
In the consciousness
For it to be known.

18
Vibrations and sounds within the consciousness
Are known when in the presence
Of the Pure and Silent Song.

19
Consciousness cannot know itself
By its own awareness.
It can only be known by the absolute awareness
Of the Pure and Silent Song.

20
Perceiver and perceived
Cannot exist together.
Consciousness must give way to the unseen worlds
Or the unseen worlds must give way to consciousness.

21

If consciousness were to experience itself
Through the workings of consciousness,
Unorganized memories would run rampant,
Bringing confusion and madness.
Awareness is the only way to experience consciousness.
It brings quiescence.

22

At the heart of this quiescence
Resides the complete knowledge of consciousness.
In the act of knowing itself through awareness,
Consciousness takes on the shape and action of awareness.

23

The Seer's new state of conscious awareness
Allows him to have a complete experience
Of the phenomenal world.
The musician manages and directs this experience
With his music.

24

Through the creativity of his music
The Seer's entire being
Serves the Pure and Silent Song
Of pure awareness.

25

When the musician can flow effortlessly
Between consciousness and pure awareness
He can see the contrast and interplay in all things.

26
When the musician can see the contrast and interplay
In all things,
He rides natural forces towards Kaivalya.

27
The Seer's devotion to music must be great
Or he will be distracted by the sights and sounds
That exist within the region between
The true and the false world.

28
These distracting sights and sounds
Can only be managed through Complete Musicianship.

29
Complete Musicianship is essential
To the final stage of Complete Release.
Without it, we would not know how to navigate
The essential natures of phenomenal experience,
Consciousness, or the light of pure awareness.
It aligns us to the Pure and Silent Song.

30
All friction and suffering,
All good and evil,
All karma and destructive passion
Is neutralized
By the Pure and Silent Song.